## Praise for *Pelvic Liberation*

"I offer Ms. Howard my profound appreciation for this book and my deep affection as a friend. I can confidently say that you will be more educated about your body, and happier and healthier, when you incorporate her suggestions into your life."

> —Judith Hanson Lasater, Ph.D., P.T.,
> yoga teacher since 1971 and author of eight books on yoga

"Insightfully and eloquently written, Leslie Howard's book combines a keen understanding of physiologic contributors to pelvic health problems in women with a holistic approach to their management. I recommend this to women of all ages."

> —Alison Huang, MD, MAS, MPhil
> Women's Health Clinical Research Center
> University of California San Francisco

"Leslie Howard is giving us a loud and important wake up call. This is an important book and it should be read by everyone."

> —Colleen Saidman Yee, author of *Yoga For Life*
> and co-founder of Urban Zen

"Leslie Howard has written a seminal book to enlighten us all about pelvic health. Ms. Howard clearly lays out... an extensive presentation of yoga poses,... how to practice them and the exact effect each pose has on the pelvic floor.... Yoga practice can offer women a unique and deeper experience... so that we can all get to know our own bodies and how truly intelligent and miraculous they are."

> —Isa Herrera, MSPT, CSCS, author of *Ending Pelvic Pain*

"Leslie has written a masterful treatment on an area of crucial concern to all women... will certainly become a classic in its field."

> —Richard Rosen, author and yoga teacher

D1160132

# Pelvic Liberation

*Using Yoga, Self-Inquiry, and Breath Awareness*
*for Pelvic Health*

## Leslie Howard

Leslie Howard
lesliehowardyoga@gmail.com
www.lesliehowardyoga.com

This book is not intended as a substitute for the medical advice of physicians. Readers should regularly consult their physician in matters relating to their health and particularly with respect to any symptoms that may require diagnosis or medical attention.

ISBN: 978-0-692-94418-9 (paperback)

First Edition

22 21 20 19 18 17 | 10 9 8 7 6 5 4 3 2 1

Book design and composition by BookMatters, Berkeley

Illustrations by Avery Kalapa

Photo renderings by Sylvia Cruz based on original photographs by Adrian Mendoza

Cover design by James Aarons

Cover art by Katarzyna Kopańska

# CONTENTS

To all of my teachers

but especially Ramanand Patel,

who has tolerated my endless questions

and conversations about yoga, philosophy,

and pelvic floors for the last 20 years

# FOREWORD

Reading the book title *Pelvic Liberation,* the droll among us might respond with the quip, "I didn't know it was in jail." But when I read this book, it became clearer and clearer to me that *indeed the female pelvis is in a kind of jail.* I learned that in today's world, the female pelvis and the health of the organs and muscles there are at the mercy of misunderstanding, mistreatment, and misdiagnosis, as well as archaic ideas about its health that pervade both the medical and lay worlds.

One of the factors that helped create this situation is the general ignorance most women have about their pelvis and all the functions that go on there. In large numbers, we are surprisingly unaware of our pelvic health and how it affects our general health; of how the pelvic floor functions during intercourse, urination, defecation, and in normal daily healthy movements of our body as a whole. The pelvic floor even plays a meaningful part in every inhalation and exhalation we experience.

Leslie Howard has written a seminal book to enlighten us all about pelvic health. Ms. Howard clearly lays out the anatomy of the pelvis and how this anatomy functions. Her description of the pelvic floor muscles, where they are and what they do, gave me excellent ways to think about their function.

All day after I read this section, I thought about my pelvic floor with new awareness and admiration. Why are we not teaching every girl, every woman, every health practitioner, regardless of gender, this information? A lot of suffering would be alleviated if the knowledge presented in this part alone were widely disseminated and understood.

But there are more jewels to be had in this book, not the least of which are the personal stories of women, including the author. These give the reader insight into the extent to which the health of the pelvis, and especially the pelvic floor, shapes our daily life and the process of pregnancy and childbirth.

I have had the pleasure of knowing Ms. Howard for decades. We first became acquainted when she studied yoga with me; we are both yoga teachers. As this acquaintance grew, we slowly evolved from teacher and student into professional colleagues. Our latest interaction has been to serve on a National Institutes of Health (NIH) study about incontinence in women and the use of yoga asana (poses) to help that condition.

One of the most useful and almost surprising points that *Pelvic Liberation* emphasizes is that there are two types of female incontinence: stress incontinence and urge incontinence. Apparently the typical instruction that we should all practice the widely taught technique commonly called Kegels can actually be a problem for those of us suffering from urge incontinence. Ms. Howard provides an excellent explanation of the difference between the two types of incontinence, and this section alone makes this book a must-have for all women. But I especially recommend this section for female yoga practitioners who may be practicing too many Kegels, as well as practicing their yoga poses in a way that makes the pelvic floor *too tight,* thus actually compromising its function.

The book ends with an extensive presentation of yoga poses, and the author explains how to practice them and the exact effect each pose has on the pelvic floor. She believes, as I do, that yoga practice can offer women a unique and deeper experience of the pelvic floor, as well as a mental attitude of self awareness that will make yoga practice more effective.

Additionally, throughout the book, she offers her readers other practices of self-discovery besides asana, so that we can all get to know our own bodies and how truly intelligent and miraculous they are.

Ms. Howard brings us a new perspective on pelvic health and shows us how much we need this information in a world where what we look like trumps what we feel like much of the time.

I offer Ms. Howard my profound appreciation for this book and my deep affection as a friend. I hope you feel the same toward her when you have finished reading *Pelvic Liberation*. I can confidently say that you will be more educated about your body, and happier and healthier, when you incorporate her suggestions into your life.

*Judith Hanson Lasater*
SAN FRANCISCO, CA
AUGUST 2017

*Judith Hanson Lasater, Ph.D., P.T., has been a yoga teacher since 1971 and is the author of eight books on yoga.*

# HOW TO USE THIS BOOK

**Self-Exploration:** Using my pelvic story as an example, *Pelvic Liberation* can take you on your own journey of self-exploration and healing.

**Healing and Treatment:** If you are reading this book, I assume that you or someone in your life is experiencing challenging issues with the female pelvis and that you are wanting a deeper understanding of your pelvis and non-invasive ways to heal what ails it. Or maybe you are a yoga teacher or healthcare practitioner who is looking for new ways to treat or improve pelvic conditions.

**Being Female in the Western World:** In Chapter I, I introduce some of the cultural contexts most women in the Western world encounter and how these contexts affect our health. I ask you, the reader, to reflect on how being female may increase the likelihood of certain experiences and how these experiences register in the body.

**Anatomy:** Chapter II is dedicated to anatomy and unhealthy versus optimal functioning of the pelvic floor. Here you can learn about over-tight or over-loose muscles and how gluteus muscles and core muscles affect the health of the pelvis.

**Maladies:** Chapter III is an overview of some of the more common conditions, cures, and misconceptions.

**Yoga and Breathing Practices:** Chapter IV explains proper breathing practices and yoga postures to help alleviate symptoms for certain conditions. Some readers will want to just skip to the yoga poses and sequences for their particular health issue. This section includes some suggested sequences for each kind of unhappy pelvis.

**Creating Community—Women to Women:** In the final chapter, I suggest introducing *Pelvic Liberation* into your women's book club. Participating in my own book club has shown me the deep bonding that happens over time and the valuable friendships and discussions that emerge as a result of our monthly meeting.

# PREFACE

Why a book about the pelvis? For one, because that's where we all start; we enter the world from our mother's womb and pelvis. The attending doctor or midwife quickly glances at our pelvis, noting if a boy or girl, and at that moment a journey begins. This book is for those of us that have a female pelvis. As girls, we are all exposed to relentless conditioning. We will be told to walk, sit, stand, move, and behave in ways that are appropriate, sexy, ladylike, and motherly and will even be told which bathroom to use. By adulthood, each of us will carry these ways of being women throughout our body, but we will feel them particularly in the pelvic region, the part of our body most deeply associated with our gender. The pelvic region becomes a complex, multilayered storage unit—I call it the original 1-800-MINI-STORAGE—the place where we store the things we can't let go of but don't want to deal with right now.

In our culture, the mental and physical geography of sexuality and elimination can seem like a forbidden land. This can lead to health issues that are both emotional and physical in nature. We need to explore and liberate this terrain and take charge of ourselves—openly acknowledge and understand our issues—and skillfully tune in to the healing power of our own bodies. For most of us, this is a departure from how our mothers' and grandmothers' generations approached pelvis-related health problems. Women have accomplished a lot in their fight for equal rights and healthcare choices; I believe it's now time to take the next step. It's time to liberate our pelvis.

~

"Every pelvis has a story" is what I tell my students. My story will unfold for you in the pages of this book.

In 2005, I had already been a yoga teacher for 20 years, so I thought I knew the anatomy and mechanics of "down there" fairly well. But around that time, I began to experience pain and discomfort in this nether region. And then as I worked to figure out why I was having pain and discomfort, I realized that much of my knowledge about the pelvic area was abstract, generic, and derived mostly from anatomy books. I didn't understand the specifics of *my* pelvis, the muscles housed within it and that entire region's relationship to the rest of my body, mind, and life history. It was as if there were a red circle/slash sign over my pelvis.

I began experimenting with yoga poses and breathing practices to familiarize myself with, and ultimately explore, the many layers of trauma, held emotion, and pain that lay hidden between my hip bones. The more I understood how the intricacies of my pelvis intersected with personal history, cultural conditioning, sexism, anatomy, and symptoms of ill-health, the more I began to see how my pelvis was tied to my general well-being—physically, emotionally, spiritually. It turned out that my pelvic floor muscles were way too tight, but I had no idea why or how that had happened. My exploration turned into an investigation of the factors that shaped me, such as my postural, sexual, and medical history, my struggles with body image, and the influence of relationships, family, culture, advertising, media, and movies.

Much of advertising, media, and the movies portray women

as sexual objects, or as incomplete without a man. I know this contributes to how I feel about my physical self and specifically my pelvis. Societal and cultural factors, familial and personal events—all of them leave an imprint, shaping the way we inhabit our bodies. Bringing the story of my pelvis to light became a key component of my evolution as a human being.

~

My goal of healing myself ultimately grew into a desire to share what I was learning. As a longtime yoga teacher, I knew the transformative power of self-awareness and the healing that comes from yoga postures and focused breathing practices. I developed a yoga protocol that eventually formed the cornerstone of my pelvic floor workshops. After leading workshops locally in the San Francisco Bay Area, I grew confident enough to pitch them to yoga studio owners around the country. Thanks to the power of women telling other women about my work, yoga studios, both nationally and internationally, began to reach out to me. Then in 2010, I received an unexpected phone call from researchers at the University of California, San Francisco (UCSF).

Women's health researchers Leslee Subak, M.D., Professor of Obstetrics, Gynecology, and Reproductive Sciences and chair of the ob/gyn department at Stanford Medical School, and Alison Huang, M.D., Associate Professor of Medicine and of Epidemiology and Biostatistics, asked me to collaborate on a study and design a yoga class to address incontinence. The study was carried out three years later in collaboration with senior yoga teacher Judith Lasater, Ph.D. Judith and I were asked to come up with a series of yoga postures that would help alleviate urinary incontinence in women age 40 and over. We designed a program of 15 postures to be practiced three times a week that would improve urinary incontinence. The pilot study, which included 18 women, resulted in a 70% overall decrease in incontinence frequency in six weeks.[1] Based on these results, we received funding from the National Institutes of Health to conduct a larger and more rigorous follow-up trial in which yoga was compared against a physical conditioning program.

I suggested that we do a study on yoga to relieve pelvic pain. I knew that yoga and breathing practices helped me with my pelvic pain, but I wanted to put both to the test. In 2014, the team received a small grant to create a therapeutic yoga program for the treatment of pelvic and genital pain in women. The study was completed in June 2016 and the results of that study showed a 42% improvement in symptoms in six weeks.

My wish is for every woman to be curious about her pelvis, to explore intimately how her pelvis works, and to heal herself. The pelvis is a rich and wondrous place to start. It is the seat of our physical selves and our sexuality; it is an area that can be charged with emotion, mystery, and taboo, the seat of bodily functions, discussion of which have often been excluded from polite conversation—excluded at a cost. Understanding and liberating the pelvis is one way we can become more fully integrated, connected human beings.

# 1 | Every Pelvis Has a Story: Exploring Historical and Cultural Stereotypes

What is the pelvic floor? Many people might respond with a shrug or a blank stare; the slightly more knowledgeable might point to "down there."

Let's say I were to ask you what part of the body is the most crucial to maintaining good posture? You might say the feet and legs, or maybe the abdominal muscles. While those parts are important, they are not our foundation, or the part of our body that integrates the head and torso with the legs and the feet. The foundation is the pelvic floor.

But the pelvic floor is more than just the bedrock that supports the rest of our "building"—it houses our energy and influences how we hold ourselves while standing, sitting, walking, or having sex. In other words, the pelvic floor is key to performing our everyday activities.

A few things we probably all know about the pelvis: It has two hip bones. And we can place our hands on these bones to convey how we feel—sexy, impatient, proud, or angry at our partner who is late for dinner.

Needless to say, there's more to the pelvis than those hip bones. The pelvic floor is a group of muscles situated at the bottom of the pelvis. These muscles are attached to the sitting bones on either side, to the pubic bone in front, and the tailbone in back. These muscles have a serious job: They hold our abdominal organs in and up. They are part of the platform for the vulva and pubic hair. They also manage what goes in and what goes out "down there," such as urination, defecation, and sexual activity. When the pelvic floor is off balance, everything on top of it—torso, shoulders, neck, head—and everything below it—groins, legs, feet—can be off balance. The pelvis provides a foundation and fulcrum for our entire bodies.

Still think of it as just a resting place for your hands?

Unfortunately, the pelvic floor is often misunderstood, or completely overlooked, by the majority of the medical and wellness community (with the exception of those pioneering physical and occupational therapists who specialize in the pelvic floor).

In the yoga world, the pelvic floor is also underappreciated. While focused on by prenatal yoga classes or schools of yoga that emphasize the pelvic floor contraction known as the "root lock" (*mula bandha*), outside of a few worthwhile articles on the pelvic floor, you won't find a lot of yoga-related books on the topic. Hence, my book. Here, I'll offer multiple perspectives on the pelvic floor—cultural, anatomical and, of course, yogic. My hope is that by sharing my experiences and explorations on the topic, you will become pelvically savvy.

Historically, we have mistreated our pelvis. We've constrained it with corsets, exaggerated it with bustles, hidden it under muumuu dresses, squeezed it into jeans, tortured it with shapewear (formerly known as girdles), and misaligned it with high heels. It gets flossed with thongs and g-strings, sweetened by lube, perfumed by intimate spray, odor neutralized by douching, and even "rejuvenated" with cosmetic surgery. It's been manicured, coiffed, and waxed. Why such mistreatment of a crucial part of our bodies?

One answer lies in one guiding principle: political control of the female pelvis by men. Western patriarchy can be read as men attempting to dominate women by controlling the pelvis and the vital organs housed within.[1] Methods include demonization—*Cover it, lest a man have temptation; skirts must extend below the knee;* erasure of the unique complexities of the female body when doing so suits the needs of medical professionals—*The doctor will tell you to give birth on your back, which is easier for* him; neutralization—*Barbie, anyone?* and ridicule—*Why do you need all that hair?!? Get rid of it!* The female pelvis is desensualized: *Quick! Cover up that smell before someone notices it!* The female pelvis is shamed: *Menstruating? Take your pain meds, hide your tampons, and be discreet!* The female pelvis is weaponized: *You are cranky today. Are you on the rag?* And, finally, the female pelvis is hyper-sexualized and constantly judged: *Check your local newsstands for ten surefire ways to please your man and which female star has been deemed overweight this week.*

So it's no wonder that women who dared to take ownership of their pelvic regions were targets for suspicion, ostracized, and feared. I think it's safe to say that men felt, and continue to feel, a deep unease about the powers of the female pelvis—after all, we have the ability to create, nurture, and deliver life into the world, if we choose, and they simply do not, despite all the advances in modern medicine.

When I started on my journey toward pelvic liberation, I wasn't initially focused on how society treats women and their bodies. Eventually, I realized that healing my pelvis required not only knowledge of yoga and anatomy, but also an enhanced aware-ness of the larger political and cultural forces that have framed our attitudes toward "down there." What started as a desire to alleviate my pain became a quest to fully inhabit and understand my body—without shame or embarrassment—and experience the sense of aliveness that flows through all my parts. It all started, inconspicuously enough, with a yoga class.

~

In 2003, I attended a class with my yoga teacher, Ramanand Patel. He gave an unfamiliar instruction: "Lift your pelvic floor!"

Now I had been practicing yoga for over 15 years but had nev-er heard this particular instruction. *Pelvic floor?* I thought. *Does he mean, "down there?" How would I "lift" it?* After class, I asked Ramanand for more details. He smiled and suggested I study with Susanne Kemmerer, a physical therapist who specializes in the pelvic floor. I signed up for one of her workshops and my pelvic floor obsession took root.

Susanne taught me that a weak and neglected pelvic floor can lead to all kinds of health issues. She introduced me to pelvic floor anatomy and taught me a variety of exercises designed to strengthen the muscles and encourage that "lift" that Ramanand mentioned. From that time, I resolved not to have a weak pelvic floor. I dedicated 15 minutes of my daily home yoga practice to the exercises Susanne had given us.

A few months later, one of my longtime students asked me about my new practice. "You have to teach me this," she implored, "Sometimes I pee in my pants. I could really benefit from this." The truth was that I didn't feel quite ready to teach women about the pelvic floor, but my student was so eager that I didn't want to let her down.

So I invited a small group of my female students to my home to discuss the pelvis. To prepare, I read every book I could find on the subject, experimented with my own yoga practice, and put together my own workshop. I taught some of what I had learned from Susanne, as well as additional insights from my readings and yoga practice. The class was well received and gave me the confidence to design my pelvic floor workshops, which I began to teach locally. I was passionate, I felt competent in the subject matter, and my students told me how much they got out of it. Everything was going swimmingly—until it wasn't.

About a year after I started my daily pelvic floor exercises, intercourse with my husband started to become painful. I was in my 40s and wondered if this was just what happens with age. Was I perimenopausal? Was it psychological? I didn't quite know what to do about it and felt isolated and embarrassed about it and so opted for the easy solution and avoided intimacy.

To make matters worse, I began experiencing pain when I spent long periods of time in the car. First, my buttocks would ache. Then I began to feel burning between my sitting bones. But unlike sex, I couldn't simply avoid driving! Something had to be done, and I tried everything I could think of. I'd lift my entire pelvis while driving, hovering over the seat as if in a dirty public bathroom; I experimented with sitting on towels, rolled up yoga mats, even a plank of wood. Nothing helped.

That's when the pelvic floor fairies sent me Lizanne Pastore, P.T., M.A., COMT. She is a pelvic floor specialist, who invited me to consult with her. Her practice includes internal examination of the vagina and palpating and massaging the pelvic floor muscles.

During our appointment, Lizanne's gentle, reassuring demeanor put me at ease. But the examination quickly went from easeful to uncomfortably enlightening as her gloved and lubricated finger slowly went inside my vagina to feel the tone of my pelvic floor. As soon as she put the slightest pressure on the deepest layer of the pelvic floor, I felt a pain so sharp that Lizanne nearly had to peel me off the ceiling. "Hypertonic pelvic floor syndrome," she diagnosed. "Your pelvic floor muscles are too tight."

I was dismayed. I didn't even know a woman *could* be too tight. What was I missing? Then tiny light bulbs started going off in my head and in my pelvis. *I think I may have done this to myself.* I told Lizanne about my daily exercises and my new mantra: "If you are female and getting older, your pelvic floor is getting saggy." She looked at me with bemusement: "The pelvic floor can be too tight, too loose, and often a combination of both." And with those words, my world changed again.

Leaving her office, I felt an extraordinary experience of levity. There was an unfamiliar sense of space "down there." I felt as if I had a beautiful peacock feather tail. After a few minutes, I also realized the pain in the right side of my neck, which I'd had for months, was gone. How was that possible? Lizanne had only massaged my pelvic floor—could that have been what made the pain stop? If so, how were the two connected? I needed to think and I went for a long walk.

My initial thoughts were that my pelvic floor muscles were too tight because I had overdone the exercises that Susanne had taught me, or I had done them incorrectly. As I pondered the source of my newly discovered pelvic tightness, memories began to rise from my more recent and distant past. I remembered that, as a little girl in the car with my father, he got angry with me every time I asked to stop so I could pee. I learned to hold it in. Eventually, I was so afraid of his anger that I didn't ask until I absolutely couldn't bear it anymore. Irritated, he would ask me to hold it until the next rest area, and when I couldn't, he became even more annoyed and I felt humiliated.

Other memories came back: How intolerable and uncomfortable tampons were for me as a teenager; my assumption that painful gynecological exams were normal; my first sexual encounter at age 15, being seduced by an older man; then, five years later, a date rape. As the memories stacked up, I saw that this series of emotionally charged events had directly impacted my pelvis. I was still holding on emotionally and physically to their collective impact. These were just a few of the many memories that returned involving me and my pelvis. Emotional trauma—even distant—can lead to chronic bracing or "holding tight" of certain muscle groups. The reasons for my excessive tightness were way more complex than overdoing a few exercises.

I felt such shame. After all, I had spent the last 15 years building my life around the body-centric practice of yoga. My community looked to me as a senior teacher with thousands of hours of training, and here I was acknowledging that I was divorced from this part of my body. I cringed thinking of the early workshops I had taught about the pelvic floor. What a disservice to my students not to have taught that the pelvic floor and its muscles could also be too tight. I had fallen for the premise that it was all about strength. However, not everybody needs strengthening exercises. People like me must learn to relax the pelvic floor muscles, to undo and unravel our habitual pattern of holding. I had to completely change my approach to the pelvis and embrace the idea that letting go can be the marker of a different type of strength.

In my next session with Lizanne, she told me that we couldn't resolve the tension in my pelvic floor muscles simply through her twice-monthly massages. Getting my bound-up muscles to soften was something I would also need to attend to on my own. I needed to learn how to massage my own pelvic floor muscles, which would facilitate faster healing. Deep down I knew that I needed to learn how to take care of myself—in more ways than one.

So Lizanne taught me how to massage my own pelvic muscles, and these hands-on techniques were one pivotal component for pain relief. However, there was a much greater healing process ahead: how could I address the issue if I didn't really understand what caused it? A single afternoon's walk had revealed a number of incidents that might have contributed to my chronic tightness, but how did I know that this wasn't just the tip of the iceberg? I needed to investigate my personal history and its cultural context.

I realized that self-empowerment was not just a means to the cure, a step on the path to physical and emotional health—it *was* the cure. Disempowerment had led to the tightening of my pelvic floor muscles in the first place. I needed to confront its manifestations in the pelvis and in my life. And with that, my *Pelvic Liberation* journey began.

~

To physically look at our pelvis we have to arm ourselves with mirrors and flashlights. To emotionally look at it, we may have to arm ourselves with courage and tissue boxes.

My first order of business was to write down all the events and influences that had impacted the way I was in my body, particularly my pelvis. Our bodies are recording devices, where a "life map" begins to take shape. We brace ourselves against trauma, anxiety, and fear. The way we sit, stand, breathe, and walk through the world is a reflection of what has happened to us. Many of the traumatic events that happened to me and my pelvis were stored away, lodged in the bands of my pelvic floor muscles, holding on for dear life. If they let go, surely the world would fall apart.

I wrote down the factors that shaped the emotional anatomy of my pelvis. I encourage you to do the same. Keeping a journal is an excellent way of exploring and shedding light on what our bodies store. When you put pen to paper, you will most likely be surprised by all the things that you and your pelvis have been through. For some of us, this first step may evoke strong emotions and possibly

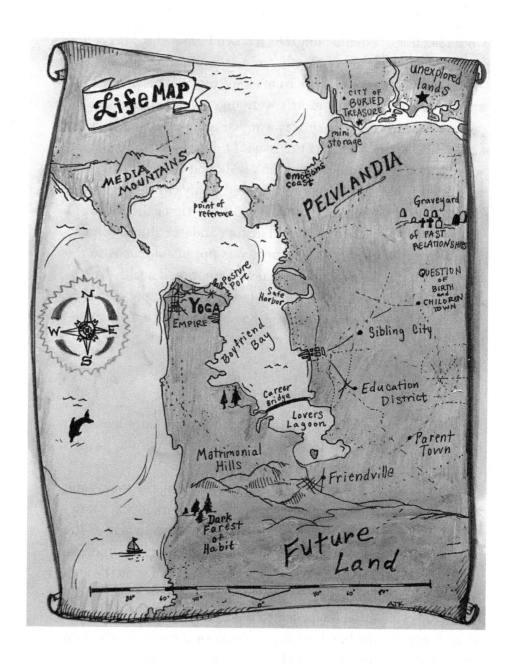

painful memories. But remember that their strength is a reflection of the strength locked away in us. To bring these issues forth and shine the light of knowledge, awareness, and compassion on them puts us on the path to self-empowerment.

## Pelvic Inquiry—The Story of Your Pelvis

The questions and suggestions below are not meant to be a template; they are neither systematic nor complete—in fact, some of them may not feel relevant to you at all. However, they emerged from my own exploration as well as those of my students. My hope is that they may serve at least as a starting point for you. I encourage you to put down on paper everything you can remember that your pelvis has been through, good or bad. I begin with one episode from "the story of my pelvis."

### *My First Period and My Mother's Response*

There was considerable excitement when the girls in my circle began their periods. I eagerly anticipated the moment that I, too, would become a member of the club. At 13, my moment came. I got my first period at school, so I couldn't wait to get home and tell my mother. Her response was not what I expected: "Well, now you are a woman. You have the monthly curse." What a letdown! I remember my excitement immediately deflating and confusion setting in. What was she talking about, "the curse"? It wasn't the only awkward, derogative term I came to know. Soon I was to learn about "being on the rag," the "crimson wave," or simply "women's trouble."

My mother then handed me a little booklet distributed by Modess, a feminine napkin manufacturer, called *How to Tell Your Daughter about Her Period.* "Let me know if you have any questions," she said as she walked out of the room. I could tell by her tone, the unspoken message was "don't ask me any questions." My mom was *not* of the hippie persuasion, but even at 13 I found her response bewildering and alienating. Some of my friends told me their mothers had sat them down to have a real conversation about their impending monthlies. One friend told me her mother called all the women in their family to celebrate her entry to womanhood (which she found mortifying). What I remember was asking, "Why am I getting the silent treatment?" The implicit message was that something shameful or embarrassing was going on.

**Pelvic Inquiry**

- What was the language around your menstrual cycle?
- When/how did you find out about menstruation?
- Do you remember any of the events around your first period and the emotions that went with them?
- How did your mother (or parents) react to your first explorations down there?
- How did that affect your own self-talk around sexuality?
- How do you feel about your monthly cycle? Is it an inconvenience and messy bother? Or do you love your connection to the lunar cycle?

## Our First Explorations "Down There" and Our Parents' Reactions

One of my students told me that when she was four years old, she was curiously exploring her nether regions. Right when she had her fingers on her vulva, her mother walked in and immediately went into a tirade. "Only bad girls do such things. Don't you ever touch yourself that way again!" My student didn't have that spontaneous memory until my workshop, and she could now see how it framed her lifelong feelings around masturbation and sex.

**Pelvic Inquiry**

- Did your parents encourage bodily exploration, did they merely tolerate it, or was it something that happened behind closed doors and in silence?
- How did you explore?
- If you did explore, what were your feelings about it? Guilt, fun, curiosity?

## Susan's Misdiagnosis: Surgery Averted

Recently at a fundraiser, I talked with a woman I'll call Susan. Susan had been diagnosed with May Thurner syndrome, a rare condition in which the left iliac vein near the pelvis is compressed by the right iliac artery, and she was scheduled to have surgery to alleviate the condition. She dreaded the procedure, but after enduring pain and numbness in her pelvis for over 10 years, she didn't think she had an alternative. I suggested she come see me for Arvigo abdominal therapy and pelvic floor yoga. Although skeptical, she agreed to see me.

While working with her, I noticed an appendectomy scar. She hadn't mentioned it on my intake and when I inquired, she immediately got tears in her eyes and told me the story behind the scar. She was just 14 years old when she had severe abdominal pain and was rushed to the hospital. "You need surgery immediately, your appendix is about to burst," a doctor pronounced. Susan gripped her mother's hand. The situation would have been frightening for anyone, but as Susan was wheeled away from her mother, she got a strong whiff of alcohol on the breath of the doctor who was about to cut into her belly. She was overcome by fear, but too young to feel confident enough to speak up, and so the surgery took place. As Susan was relating the story, she realized that it was soon after that surgery that her troubles with her pelvis began.

After her appointment with me, I referred her to a pelvic floor physical therapist who discovered the misdiagnosis: She did not have May Thurner Syndrome and did not need surgery. She had hypertonic pelvic floor muscles, due in part to her past trauma. She is now pain-free.

**Pelvic Inquiry**

- Do you have any stories of being in the presence of a healthcare practitioner and not feeling heard, respected, or understood?

- How did you feel when you visited the gynecologist for the first time?

- Were there any doctor visits that made you feel uncomfortable in any way?

- Have any of your doctors asked what was going on in your life or what your stress level was at the time of your appointment?

### Sexual Trauma in My Teens

At age 15, a friend of the family who was a much older man seduced me. I was clearly not ready for sex, but I didn't have the wisdom or the courage to follow my own internal intimacy clock. Five years later, while attending college, my ex-boyfriend, who could not accept the breakup, secretly followed me as I was walking to my home. He grabbed me, threw me to the ground, held me down, and raped me. As is common with rape victims, I blamed myself for what happened. I told myself that I should have managed the breakup differently. I made excuses for him. Because I knew him, it was difficult to label this rape, and so I didn't tell anyone what had happened. Only years later was I able to see it for what it was.

### Pelvic Inquiry

- Have there been other moments that you felt somebody else took control over your body?

- What were your first sexual experiences like?

- Have you ever been sexually violated, and how did it affect you both physically and emotionally? How did it change how you related to your body?

- Did you feel any shame or guilt around them?

### A Gift from Her New Husband: An STD

A friend of mine who suffers from chronic pelvic pain attended my workshop and confided in me. Unlike her husband, she had waited until marriage to have sex. Soon after she had sex with him, she experienced searing pain in her vaginal area. Having no idea what was happening to her, she went to see a gynecologist and was diagnosed with genital herpes. She was angry with her husband for not telling her. She was hurt and felt let down and betrayed by her partner.

When the herpes virus is active, urination can be very painful. It causes extreme nerve pain in the buttocks and legs. Even though she has the virus under control with medication, her pain sometimes returns. She also has "shy bladder syndrome," meaning she cannot urinate if someone else is in the restroom. She simply can't relax her pelvic floor and urethra enough to "go."

### Pelvic Inquiry

- Have you unwittingly received an STD from a partner whom you love(d)?

- Do you have or have you had an STD? How did it affect you physically and emotionally?

- What feelings did you have after being diagnosed?

- Did you have a supportive partner or friend to share your feeling? Have you been diagnosed with any disease that is centered in the pelvis; i.e., cervical, ovarian, or uterine cancer, endometriosis, interstitial cystitis, irritable bowel syndrome? If so, were you able to get a diagnosis early, or did you have to visit more than one doctor?

- What was your support network when you were diagnosed?

### *My Partner and My Pelvis*

At my third appointment with my physical therapist, Lizanne suggested I get my husband involved in my healing process. She proposed inviting him to the next session so she could help guide him in how to massage my pelvic floor. "Um, I'm not sure if he would be willing to do that." Lizanne simply replied, "Why don't you ask him?" I did. He was up for it and suggested that I teach him. My heart filled with hope.

Prior to this, sex had become increasingly painful and challenging for my partner and me. Shielding him from the truth, I told myself this was *my* problem when in fact it was rooted in my earlier traumatic sexual experiences. I isolated myself with feelings of low self-esteem and self-blame. I developed silent strategies for avoiding sex. I would go to bed early, put my baggiest pajamas on, and never let him see me getting dressed or undressed. I became not only sex averse, but also affection averse. I thought, "Oh I'd better not be affectionate, I don't want him to get his hopes up." Unfortunately, this is an all too common attitude for women that can easily lead to disaster. When we begin avoiding affection, the end of the relationship may not be far behind.

At first I felt embarrassed and shy. Yet we had enjoyed a good sex life before my pelvic pain started and this helped give me the courage to invite him in. To my surprised delight, he was really open about it and he wanted to learn. It felt like we were on a bit of an adventure together. One of my symptoms, which was a total bummer, was that when I had an orgasm, it hurt. My pelvic muscles were so tight that the contractions that most of us strive to attain and enjoy were something I tried to avoid. When I shared this with my husband, he came up with a plan; when I felt close to an orgasm, he suggested, let's stop, try to relax my pelvic floor, and then try again. It was a brilliant idea that soon enabled me to enjoy a pain free orgasm.

My persnickety pelvis was also insisting that intercourse, at least for the time being, had to be done slow, slow, slow. Now most of us know that this is not how some men approach sex. But if my husband wanted to have sex, he had to slow down. Otherwise, intercourse was painful. He was open to that too. Of course he didn't want to hurt me and it was the only way we could have penetrative sex. But because of this necessity, something really wonderful developed: We both started thoroughly enjoying this new way to make love. Our new motto became, "How slow can we go?" This was an incredible turn of events for my healing process. No longer did I feel isolated. The whole situation had been reframed as a "we" issue. It increased our intimacy level dramatically.

I tell you this incredibly personal story to encourage those of you with partners to bring them into the process. My partner was highly motivated to help me, to be involved, and he was curious. We joked regularly that his commodity value had increased greatly with his newfound knowledge of the female pelvis.

## Pelvic Inquiry

- If you are in a relationship, how much of your story or your symptoms have you shared with your partner?

- If you have confided in them, what has their reaction been?

- Do you feel supported around this issue, or have you treated it as only your problem?

- How do you feel about inviting your partner into the healing process?

### *Elvis and My Pelvis—Some Good Times*

Of course I, like most women, had many early experiences with my pelvis, experiences where I felt connected, embodied, alive—for instance when I was seven and discovered Elvis Presley. I spent countless hours in my basement playing his records over and over, dancing wildly. I remember moving my body without any inhibition, every cell burning with aliveness. I was moving my pelvis to Elvis. Of course, I had no idea of the controversy and outrage Elvis' style had provoked; to me, his gyrations seemed fun. Maybe we could all use a little more Elvis in our pelvis.

## Pelvic Inquiry

- What experiences, events, or activities do you remember in which your pelvis was directly involved that filled you with boundless energy and joyous unbridled aliveness? Playing sports? Dancing? Swimming or skinny dipping in a lake? Soaking in a hot bath? Having good sex? A beautiful birth?

It's important we understand the impact of traumatic events; but it's equally important to know and be able to identify when our bodies are relaxed and energized.

## Cutting through Stereotypes

My first forays into my personal history left me with two realizations: my pelvis had endured a lot, and I wasn't alone in this. The more I looked at what had happened to me, the more I understood the extent to which my own personal experience exemplifies larger trends in our society, with roots in our cultural history. My feeling of helplessness and humiliation in the gynecologist's chair is part of a centuries-long history of medicine and science. My traumatic rape experience is common, unfortunately, to many women worldwide. Many of the factors that shape the way we inhabit our bodies are neither random nor isolated, and our trauma is symptomatic of deeper cultural and historical factors.

Given the breadth and depth of this topic, I cannot come close to doing it justice here. And yet, I think it's important for us to at least acknowledge how pelvic health is not separate from larger cultural, historical, and political contexts. In the next section I focus especially on three areas that have a direct influence on our pelvic region and our identity as women: the female body in the beauty industry, the Western medical world, and Western gender dynamics.

### *The Beauty Industry*

> As far as cosmetics are used for adornment in a conscious and creative way, they are not emblems of inauthenticity: it is when they are presented as the real thing, covering unsightly blemishes, disguising a repulsive thing so that it is acceptable to the world that their function is deeply suspect. The women who dare not go out without their false eyelashes are in serious psychic trouble.
>
> —GERMAINE GREER, *The Female Eunuch*

The fashion industry is a $250 billion dollar conglomerate that tells us ladies how to dress and work with what we've got . . . and we all know its more about how you look than how you feel, right?

Fashion culture has a huge influence on the garments we purchase, what we think looks good, and how we adorn and move our pelvises out in the world.

The physical constraints imposed by the fashion industry touch only the surface of a layered and complex phenomenon. On the catwalk, anorexic models walk like robotic aliens, their pelvises pushed forward, teetering in high heels. The body's natural form is re-shaped, along with its movements. France has begun to outlaw the use of ultra-thin models whose extreme skinniness could be outright health-corrupting.[2] As girls, we were told how to sit appropriately: as women, we are shown how to walk sexily, tilt our heads playfully, glance seductively, and so on.

From top to toe, from hip to lip, every area of a woman's body is subject to scrutiny by the fashion and beauty police. Ideally, a healthy fashion industry would help to enhance our authentic beauty and design clothes that accentuate and celebrate the many forms of the female body, similar to how wrapping paper adorns a gift. However, many of our clothes are designed to forcefully mold, form, and coerce our bodies into something they are not. True, we no longer subject ourselves to the unhealthy compression of our organs and impaired respiration caused by wearing tight-laced steel-boned corsets that literally squeezed the life out of women for centuries. But not so fast, the corsets of old may still be with us. I vividly remember lying on my bed as a teenager, sucking in my belly as hard as I could in order to force the zipper of my skinny jeans to close. One friend told me that in the mid-70s she used to soak her jeans in water and then let them dry on her legs and butt to make them even tighter.

The serious health effects of tight pants are well studied.[3] Tight pants cause poor posture and eventually a host of problems associated with being habitually misaligned and not breathing fully. In more serious instances, however, it can also cause spinal damage, nerve compression, and muscle degradation. If we then bring our constricted and compressed package into an asymmetrical posture by putting a cell phone in one of the tight back pockets, injury is nearly guaranteed.

And if you really want to prove to yourself (and the world) that you are willing to suffer for beauty, complement your skinny jeans with some high heels. I recommend stilettos. They will not only destabilize your already constricted lower body, but, if worn frequently enough, can lead to hyperextension of the knee, ankle sprains, bunions, and hammertoes.

From tight belts to ill-fitting bras to oversized handbags, there is hardly a fashion article that hasn't willfully attempted to distort the body's natural form and alignment. And what can't be squeezed or twisted into shape can always be lifted, tucked, cut, sucked, filled up, chemically smoothed, or transplanted. According to annual statistics on plastic surgery procedures, 15.9 million surgical and minimally invasive cosmetic procedures were performed in the U.S. in 2015.[4]

Just as the corsets of old squeezed the life out of victimized torsos, so do modern beauty images squeeze and suck the self-confidence out of many who do not meet their standards. One might think that the creation of permanent dissatisfaction was indeed the industry's main objective. It exerts an immense psychological pressure on our emotional and physical bodies and in extreme cases has driven teenage girls to suicide. The dejected mood swings of young women can be easily dismissed as typical teenage behavior, usually followed by a note about hormonal imbalance. And yet, today we know much about the toll we pay for trying to be beautiful.

Fashion is big business and, sadly, it's more often about profit than healthy fit. Wouldn't it be great if the fashion industry employed physical therapists, M.D.s, and chiropractors to consult on healthy clothing choices? We need to bring awareness to our clothing choices and their impact on our posture and our health.[5] Don't get me wrong, I love dressing up and down and under and over and sexy, and I want to look my best just as much as the next person. But I don't think that we should have to shorten our breath, cut off blood flow, or squeeze and pinch our organs in the name of being trendy fashionistas.

## Men in White Coats
## and the Appropriation of the Female Pelvis

**Feminism is the radical notion that women are people.**

—MARIE SHEAR

When I was 45 years old, I was diagnosed with fibroids on and in my uterus. Fibroids are non-cancerous tumors that often cause constant discomfort and bloating in the lower abdomen (as was the case with me). I had just changed healthcare plans and my new gynecologist was a man in his 60s. At my first meeting with him, he examined me, pushed back on the stool he was perched on, and asked matter-of-factly, "Are you done having children?" I felt a sense of unease but wasn't quite sure where he was going with this line of questioning. He continued: "If so, I think you should have a hysterectomy. Your uterus has a number of fibroids, and if you aren't planning to have children, you don't really need it anymore."

I was so taken aback that my response came without thinking: "If you are done having children, should we just take out your sexual organs?" Needless to say, our appointment ended there. I found another doctor who removed the fibroids without taking my uterus too.

The idea that my uterus had but one function is a view from the early 20th century. This view is rapidly changing and instead the uterus is rightly viewed as having multiple functions: reproduction, structural integrity, sexual pleasure. However some doctors in some areas of the country still adhere to this outmoded view from 100 years ago, that the uterus's only function is to support reproduction. It's important that we remind doctors who are stuck in outdated views that their field has changed for the better. Let's take a look at other treatments involving the uterus, childbirth, and prenatal care.

Worldwide, the U.S. ranks 27th when it comes to infant mortality.[6] We have the most expensive maternity care among the industrialized nations, yet outcomes for live births rank among the worst. In the U.S., out of 4 million births per year, 98% are in hospitals and many are either medically induced or artificially stimulated.[7] You might think all this medical intervention would reduce birth-related health issues and ensure great birth experiences. In fact, the opposite is true: the massive numbers of interventions have led to high numbers of pre-term babies, infant and mother mortality, post-partum stress, and a whole battery of other complications. The World Health Organization estimates that a C-section could be considered appropriate for 10–14% of all births today.[8] The U.S. has a C-section rate hovering around 30%, up from about 4.5% in the mid-60s.[9]

Sometimes it seems that childbirth has become but a cog in the wheels of the medical machinery. Although things are changing to some degree, something is not right when medical professionals are the lead actors who drive the action and women giving birth have mere supporting roles.

Then there's what I call "hysterectomy hysteria." The U.S. has the questionable honor of having the highest hysterectomy rate in the world. About 600,000 uteruses are removed annually—that's more than one every single minute of the year.[10] During the time it takes you to get up and make tea, another five wombs have been removed.[11] Please note, there are valid reasons for a hysterectomy, such as a cancer diagnosis or metastasis, severe prolapse, or excessive bleeding. Additionally, some women have told me that their quality of life was vastly improved by the procedure.

The problem is that women are sometimes encouraged to "just have it taken out" if something doesn't seem quite right and if childbearing is no longer desirable. A 2015 University of Michigan–led study of nearly 3,400 women in Michigan shows that one in five who underwent a hysterectomy may not have needed it.[12]

In the not too recent past the womb was treated as if it were simply disposable. A hysterectomy can lead to a loss of physical sensation, loss of sexual desire, painful intercourse, a feeling of the vagina being shortened, incontinence, and an increase in pelvic floor problems.[13] Students have shared with me that post-hysterectomy, they've experienced a change in their sense of iden-

### Ode to the Womb

You will notice that throughout the book, I use the words *uterus* and *womb*. I want to say a little more about these terms.

Let's take a moment and reflect upon the difference between talking about the *uterus* and talking about the *womb*. Both share the same anatomical reference, however each has its own sense. The poet Tony Hoagland writes that "language uses us / the way that birds use sky," and that "when you say a word / you enter its vocabulary / it's got your home address, your phone number/and it won't forget."* We experience what Hoagland is saying when we talk about the womb. The sense of *uterus* conveys nothing but a medical term for a specific organ. The sense we have with *womb*, however, is of life, nature, creation, sacredness, and wisdom. The name of Delphi, site of ancient Greece's most famous oracle, is likely derived from *delphus* (womb), an archaic honoring of Earth Goddess Gaia.

*Giving birth* is used not only for childbirth, but also for any new beginning. For example, we talk about the birthplace of a culture or an idea. Similarly, womb is not just the place where babies are carried; rather, it has become synonymous with the place from which creation springs.

I think there is value in using our language consciously, with awareness of its rich connotations. When we become conscious of how we use language we increase our ability to channel the powerful energies that language carries. These energies connect us—not just to women throughout history, but also to the birthing of life and history itself.

*"Hearings" from *Donkey Gospel* (Graywolf Press, February 1998)

tity, and that if they had been fully informed of the procedure's potential side effects, they may not have opted for it.

The womb is not just a warm place to create a human. One of its many important other jobs is to provide structural integrity. The womb serves as the centerpiece of the pelvis, directly supporting both bladder and rectum and giving important support to all the organs above it. Think of it this way: if you remove some bricks from the foundation of a building, the building might not fall down but it will be less stable.

The womb also does a bit of a dance when sexually aroused.

Sex researchers Masters and Johnson reported that during various phases of sexual excitement, the uterus fills with blood and lifts up into the pelvis. Then, with further stimulation, it widens and expands, taking part in the rhythmic contractions caused by orgasm.[14] The womb is connected to many things, physical, emotional, and sensual. Choosing to have a hysterectomy is not an easy decision, but we need to be better informed of the possible adverse effects.

Common sense gives us strong signals that we should be cautious about hysterectomies and removal of the ovaries; why does the practice continue at such a high rate in the U.S.?

### What History Can Tell Us

The current attitudes in the medical community about childbirth and hysterectomies can be seen as part of a long and complex history of male appropriation of the female body. The Greek physician Galen of Pergamon (born AD 130) stated, "Women have exactly the same organs as men, but in exactly the wrong places." We now know how ridiculous this sounds, but it shows that, since a very long time ago, the male body has been taken as the norm and the female body as some deficient variation of it.

Despite their supposed physical deficiencies, there is plenty of historical evidence that shows women have traditionally been the healers in their communities and tribes since ancient times.[15] However, this started to change in the Western world as we entered the modern era. By the 14th century, men were taking over the healer roles, as evidenced by a declaration of Christian patriarchs: "If a woman dare to cure without having studied, she is a witch and must die."[16] We know that many of the women who were prosecuted and killed for "witchcraft" were, in fact, herbalists and healers from the peasant class. But the male takeover of the medical field was so successful that from the 18th century on, most midwives were men.

Just as many religions established their power through claiming moral authority over sexuality, men sought to cement their power by claiming control over women's bodies. This was made possible partly through a range of simplistic, reductive assumptions such as "sex is for procreation," and "the womb is for childbearing."[17] Not only do such functional reductions of the female body derive from predominantly male perspectives, they also undercut a woman's ability to act as an integral, self-empowered being who makes her own decisions about her own body.

Unfortunately, while our current medical model has made some significant advances in women's reproductive health issues, such as the development of safe, effective methods of birth control and safer ways to terminate pregnancy, it still has its roots in this history. If we want to cultivate a fuller view of what it is to be a woman, we need to insist on better care from the medical establishment, be more informed about our pelvic health, and look at our relationship to our pelvis. From there, better health, women's empowerment, and a richer and more fulfilling sexuality can follow.

**Pelvic Inquiry**

- What was your attitude toward doctors when you were growing up?

- Have you ever felt a conflict between common sense and medical advice?

- Have your interactions with medical professionals increased your knowledge, curiosity, and decision-making abilities, or have these professionals "taken over"?

- Have you noticed whether you internalize any of the implicit notions and values, such as feeling less valued as a woman postmenopause or post hysterectomy?

- How would you rate your trust in your body's natural intelligence and healing powers vs. medical observation and your doctor's advice?

### *Posture, or Why Wonder Woman Doesn't Tuck Her Tail*

An image, we are told, is worth a thousand words. Our body language produces several thousand such images every minute, making it an incredibly powerful means of communication. Facial expressions, gestures, the way we stand, sit, and move, all give information about thoughts, feelings, and intentions. I think we all know the embarrassing side of this truth from the awkward photos we always wanted to see removed from the family photo album! Some of the body language's "vocabulary" seems hardwired in us, such as raising an arm as a sign of triumph. Others are culturally conditioned, such as raising our middle finger as a sign of, well, you know of what. As a matter of actual fact, the ancient Greeks already used this gesture, so maybe it's more hardwired than we might assume.

We all know that body language is an important part of how we communicate with others; but recent research reveals how much body language also communicates to the self. It not only tells others about who we are, but it in turn shapes the way we think and feel about ourselves.

A core element of our body language is posture. The posture we assume at any given moment is an expression of what *is* happening to us as well as what *has* happened to us. One person might look "beaten down by life." Another has a "chest bursting with pride." I remember visiting my grandmother, who would always greet me with her arms up in a V-position, the visible manifestation of joy and her readiness to scoop me up. As a child, nobody had to explain that posture to me, I just knew what it meant.

Many of our society's most common activities are inscribed into our body language as postures. When a student comes to see me for pelvic pain, my first question usually is "What do you do all day? Do you sit, stand, or walk for work? Do you drive a car for many hours a day?" Next I'll ask her to show me how she sits. Ten times out of ten, the student is sitting on her tail. Then I might inquire about what is going on in her life, "Is anything particularly stressful happening? What are your most dominant emotions?"

Our posture lies right at the intersection of the factors that shape the way we are in our bodies and how we respond to these factors.

Let's take a look at a normal day in many a woman's life with a character named Rosie Roundback. Rosie gets up between 5 and 6 AM to get herself and the kids ready for the day. She fixes breakfast (probably at a kitchen counter that's a bit too low for her), packs the kids' bags (bending over several times), shuffles them into the car (lifting, bending, and twisting), and drives them to school and then herself to work (getting stuck in rush hour). She grabs another coffee and then sits down at her desk, where she will remain slumped in front of a computer screen until lunch time . . . By now, you probably know where the story is going. Rosie sits all day, picks up her kids, bends, twists, slumps, gets stuck in traffic again, cooks, cleans—and finally plops down on the couch to watch an hour or two of TV before crashing in bed and sleeping in a fetal position for the next eight hours. This is a grueling routine for many a pelvis in the U.S.

Now, add to the physical stress a few emotional ingredients. Rosie's boss calls her out in front of her peers; being put on the spot to speak publicly makes her very uncomfortable, and so she internally cringes, wanting to disappear. At home, she has a phone call with her ex-husband about child support, and she feels—once again—her entire body tensing. To get herself in a better mood, she puts on a sexy pair of high heels and meets up with a few friends at the local bar where she sits cross-legged and round-shouldered; after a few drinks, she leans onto the table, doubled over with sadness.

The physical and emotional toll our bodies pay for our lifestyle is encoded in our postures. The postures, in turn, influence the way we think and feel about ourselves. A famous study by Amy Cuddy even claimed that postures that are considered "high power"—think Wonder Woman's stance—boost testosterone and lower cortisol.[18] Really, can you picture Wonder Woman tucking her tail or slumping in a chair?

*Posture,* after all, is both a noun and a verb. Just look at the various roles each of us might play throughout our lives as career woman, working mom, nurturing mom, sexy spouse, and so on. Each of these roles tends to require a different set of postures, such as looking strong, looking cute, looking understanding. How any given posture affects our health is usually considered no more relevant than the list of possible side effects in tiny print on the side of your bottle of aspirin. But in fact, as we'll find out later in this book, our habitual postures as we go through the day can have a serious impact on our health, our level of energy, and our perception of self.

## Pelvic Inquiry

- In your mind, go over your typical day. What different postures do you habitually take?

- How do you sit at the computer desk, in the car, at the kitchen table?

- How do the emotional stresses of your various roles affect your posture? What body language do you have that is influenced by your familial role models?

- What is the body language of your mother, your sisters, or your children? How has your body language changed over time? Is it the same today that it was when you were in high school?

- Are you even conscious of when you are "posturing" today? We are so used to the habitual ways of moving our bodies that it can be difficult to even know what postures we are assuming and when. Maybe ask a good friend how she or he sees your body language, or look over some photos.

## *Tall Tails*

I happen to be a cat lover. I've learned a lot about the profound connection between emotion and self-expression and posture from my favorite felines, and if you knew my cat Griffin, you would understand why. It's fascinating how many emotions Griffin expresses with his tail.

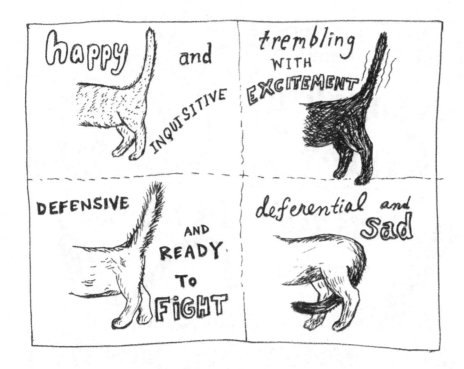

Humans are no less expressive than cats—except that our forms of expression are usually either stifled or transformed by cultural conventions. The remnant of our once high-flying tails, the coccyx or tailbone, was not meant to be a weight-bearing bone; it should have freedom to move. However, take a quick look around your local coffee shop and you will see most folks sitting with a curved lower back, tucking their tailbones between their legs.

When I looked at my own posture during my pelvic pain odyssey, I discovered that I was tucking my tail all of the time. I coined a nickname for myself (and many of my friends): I am a recovering *mothertucker.*

### Pelvic Inquiry

- We are a nation of mothertuckers. How do you think that might affect us psychologically?

- If you could wish yourself a tail or just imagine that you had one, what would it look like? I have come up with the following "tail chart" (please note this is just for fun). What does your choice of tail say about you?

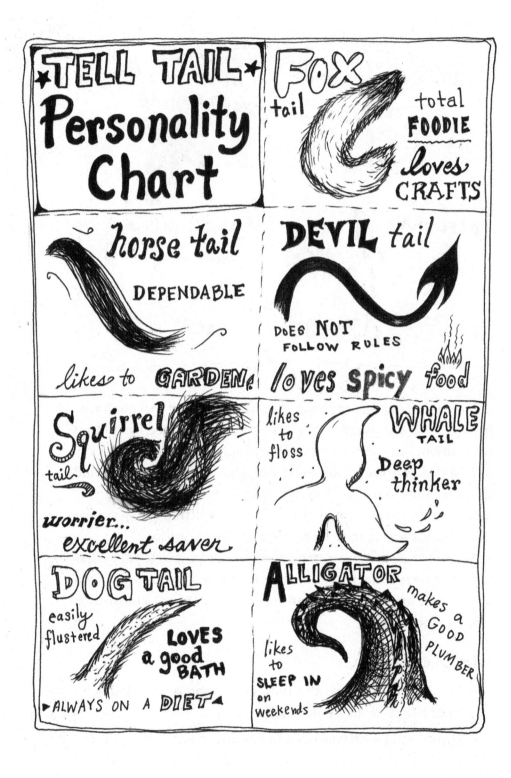

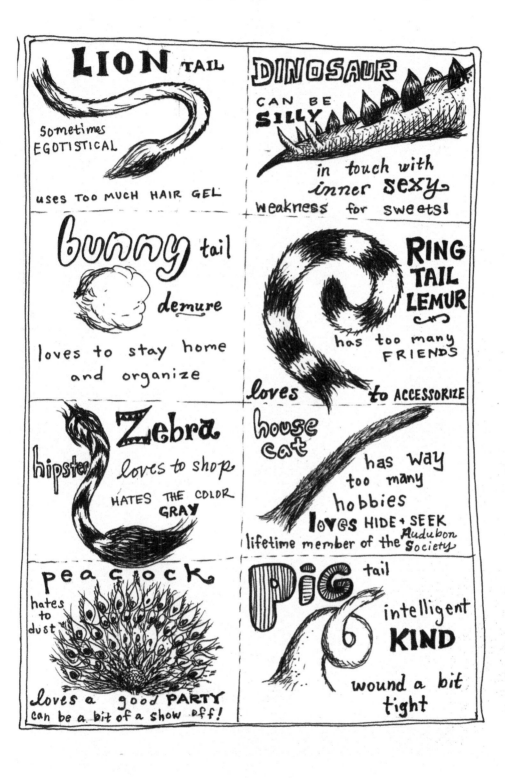

# 11 | Noble Anatomy: The Magic of Pelvlandia

When I stood before her, this unknown woman in repose, I saw myself, my mother, my grandmother, a woman revealed lovingly by a man's hand and eye . . . I wept. I wept at the beauty of naming it so clearly. *Origin of the World*. We come into this world through women, a woman who is spent, broken open, in awe. No wonder women have been feared and worshipped ever since man first saw the crowning of a human head here, legs spread, a brushstroke of light.

—TERRY TEMPEST WILLIAMS,
"When Women Were Birds: Fifty-Four Variations on Voice"
(on Gustave Courbet's painting, *L'Origine du monde*)

## What the Heck Is "Down There"?

Confucius famously observed that we learn wisdom in three ways: first, by reflection (the noblest); second, by imitation (the easiest); and third, by experience (the bitterest). Those immortal words should have been spoken with the female pelvis in mind. After all, we often start learning about the pelvic muscles when we are experiencing pain and discomfort—clearly the bitterest way. Some of us, however, go to workshops and learn by following a teacher—arguably the easiest (depending on whose workshops you take). And only a third rarified group gains pelvic wisdom through reflection, to be more precise: through reflecting on its anatomy. What we will be reflecting on next is the female anatomy. Hence, we may call the resulting knowledge "noble anatomy."

Anatomical knowledge is power. And learning anatomy from books is a good thing to do. But the practice of yoga (and other body practices) gives you the opportunity to learn anatomy *experientially*. The word anatomy refers to the science of both the body's structure and its internal workings. Understanding both is critical to making informed and empowered medical decisions. It is not the only foundation to base our decisions on, but it is a necessary one.

A clear understanding of our pelvis's anatomy greatly facilitates the self-exploration of our body and expands the experiential knowledge we can gain. We can much more easily identify what we have words for. What we see when we take out the mirror, what we make out by feeling with our fingers, and what we sense when we move our muscles—all that becomes more distinct and focused when we have the anatomical language to name *what* we are looking at, feeling, moving, and so on. Cognitive knowledge (words) and experiential knowledge (feeling and sensation) can be strong supports to each other. The ability to conceptualize what can't be seen often helps us to experience it.

Maybe best of all, only when we understand the anatomy of the pelvis do we come to fully appreciate and admire its beauty and miraculous powers. A few years ago, I attended a cadaver lab class with a brilliant teacher, Gil Hedley, and had the chance for a firsthand look at a womb and a sacrum. It was a profound, life changing experience.

Since our corpse had a body as long and lithe as a gazelle, our group named her *Gisele*. Gisele was a tall, thin 79-year-old who looked much younger than her age, even as she was lying on the steel table, filled with embalming fluids. Over the course of several days, we carefully removed layer after layer, veil after veil of skin and membranes, until our student team finally got to the organs. I remember my utter amazement at how small her uterus was; the uterus shrinks post-menopause, but this one was *tiny*. We marveled at the fimbriae (Latin for "fringe") of the fallopian tubes. To me, they looked like little fingers, and I imagined them doing a little come hither dance with great focus and intent to entice the egg and help it on its journey to the womb. The fimbriae are as delicate as petals on a flower.

After admiring the uterus for a good long while, I lifted my scalpel and began to carefully detach it. Goose bumps popped up on my legs. This small jewel was the way through which *every* human being on this planet had come into existence. Somehow holding this small womb in the palm of my hand connected me to everyone.

On the last day of our lab, there was not much left of Gisele, but my amazement didn't wane. We had gotten down to her bones, and I admired the beautiful shape and color of the pelvic bones and sacrum. Most of us have seen plasticized models of skeletons, but the beauty of real bone is simply mesmerizing. It has a gray tone with a translucent quality and swirls of polychromatic grays . . . absolutely beautiful. Next up for the group was to explore how the sacroiliac joint works.

When the sacrum was freed from the ilium, a collective "ahh" sound ran through the lab. It seems that I wasn't the only one for whom it was a special moment. I wanted to hold it in my hand. When I did I was surprised by the disparity between the light physical weight and the heavy emotional weight. At lunch that day we had debated whether there was still any spirit in our cadaver. My first reaction had been, "No, of course not." But as I held this gorgeous sculpted bone in my hands, I wondered. The sacrum is a witness to all that goes on in the pelvis. As we bend forward, it nods its upper body in agreement, and as we lie down to rest, it provides a platform for the lower organs to rest upon. In times of trial, the sacrum bears witness to painful periods, awkward encounters with sexuality, and, tragically, sometimes to sexual abuse. In the best of times, the sacrum bears witness to the waxing and waning of a woman's moon cycle, to creativity, passion, love, and the blossoming of a future human. In later years, it presides over a woman's transition to cronedom.

~

In the following section is a guide to the physical territory of "Pelvlandia." We will begin with the bones, move on to the organs, and then look at the muscles. My hope is that you study this map with curiosity and compassion in your heart. If your pelvis currently has "issues," it's only letting you know that something is not working in your life—be it physical, spiritual, emotional, or a combination of all. Let's make friends with our pelvis and enjoy the magic of noble anatomy.

### Bones, Muscles, Organs

#### Bones

Our ability to walk upright is often put forward as one of the most distinctive features of being human, along with our massive brains, our propensity to make tools, our capacity for self-reflection, and, I may add, our unique ability to accessorize. But seriously, only humans among animals have developed an upright walk. All other primates are basically quadrupedal, that is, they walk on all fours. Walking on two limbs may have deprived us of many fun and useful abilities, such as climbing trees at amazing speed. But it's also freed our hands to hold tools and carry food over great distances, features that were absolutely crucial for our evolution.

The core design that enables this feat is our pelvic structure, that complex of bones that not only connect the torso with the limbs, but also provide attachments for the muscles that support and balance the trunk. A recent article in the *New York Times* reported on studies of a highly unusual cave-dwelling fish in Thailand.[1] This creature has become an object of scientific attention because it is thought to be in the midst of an evolutionary transition, from being a fish to becoming a tetrapod or land vertebrate. Formally a swimmer, this fish is developing the ability—and the necessary anatomical features—to walk on land. A key to enabling the creature to move over solid ground, as well as swim, is its pelvis, which has adapted by joining the hind limbs, which formerly served only as fins, to the spine, so that they can serve as legs. Observe evolution in motion.

Now, I must admit that I have often wondered what on earth might have motivated our earliest ancestors to abandon their free-floating lifestyle in the oceans and instead move to land, where they had to schlep around their cumbersome body weight.

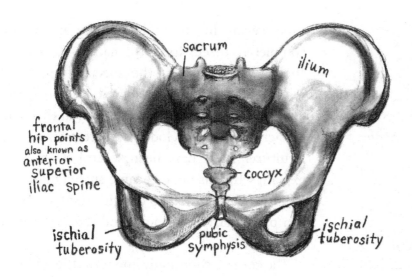

Nostalgia aside, the bone structure of the pelvis is a truly marvelous feat of engineering. Let's take a closer look at it.

The pelvis, Latin for "basin," is made up of four bones. The largest structure is made from the two hip bones, which look like giant flat ears. They consist of three parts, the ilium (plural: ilia; the ears proper), the ischium (plural: ischia; the ear lobes, so to speak; better known as the sitting bones), and the pubis bone. Broadly speaking, the main function of the hip bones is to connect the spine with the lower limbs.

Hinged between them in back is the sacrum, and at the bottom of the sacrum is our tail. Anybody who has had sacroiliac pain knows that there is movement between the ilium and the sacrum; hence it's considered a joint. Ideally, the sacrum sits nicely and symmetrically suspended between the two sides of the ilium. However, a number of factors, like poor postural habits, falls or injuries, asymmetrical activities, and so on can take it out of balance; one side may lean in a little deeper, with the other gapping and causing pain.

The sacrum is an amazing piece of art. It's the shape of a triangle and sits at the bottom of our spine. It consists of five vertebrae that are initially separated but start fusing around age 16. By the

In many East Asian practices, the lower *dan tien* (located in the lower belly, often translated as "field of elixir") is considered an area of sanctity; it is sometimes called the *hara*. The practices are about balancing the ascending and descending energy by learning how to move it up the back and down the front of the body in a complete circle (the snake swallowing its tail); this is known as the microcosmic orbit. East Asian traditions use the word *elixir* where in yogic texts it is called *kundalini* energy. Yoga practitioners are encouraged to awaken the energy and to raise it up the spine.

time we are in our mid-30s, they are usually completely fused. Its Latin name—*os sacrum,* "holy bone"—hints at the special importance many cultures have attributed to it. Already ancient Egypt appears to have revered this bone as sacred to Osiris, God of resurrection and agriculture. There have been several attempts to explain why this bone became such a dignitary. Most probably, it has to do with the fact that it is a particularly hard bone and the very last to disintegrate.

The coccyx, commonly known as the tailbone, sits at the very bottom portion of the spine, at the end of the road, so to speak. I always liked the name *coccyx*, it comes from the Greek word for the "beak of a cuckoo bird," and if you look at it from the side, it does indeed look like a beak (though I am not sure that it necessarily looks like that of a cuckoo). It consists of three to five mostly fused segments, the largest of which articulates with the lowest sacral segment. Originally, the tailbone was thought to be just one solid bone. But we now know that there are fibrous joints and ligaments between its segments that allow for some limited movement; the normal range of motion for the tailbone is around 12–14°.

Despite its small size, the coccyx has several Amazonian functions. It is not only the insertion site for multiple muscles, ligaments, and tendons; it also provides positional support to the anus. Now, as if that wasn't enough, over the last few decades the poor guy has been burdened with another major task that was definitely not in his original job description: bearing weight when humans sit in a slouchy position. Most people in our culture do that all the time, and it seems that the sitting bones have successfully outsourced their sitting duties to the tail. The structure of the tailbone was not designed to be weight bearing and for optimum health of the spine, we should not be sitting on it.

## Muscles

The pelvic floor is made up of three muscle groups. Each of these groups comprises a distinct layer that itself consists of 5–6 bands (for a total of 16). Ideally (i.e., in a healthy body), these bands all work seamlessly together, within each layer and among all three. When that's the case, they are like an incredibly strong, elastic trampoline that stretches from the tailbone to the pubic bone (back to front) and from one sitting bone to the other (side to side).

The pelvic floor muscles have a whole range of important functions: from supporting the pelvic floor organs to stabilizing connecting joints; from assisting in urinary and fecal continence to aiding in sexual performance (think orgasm); from facilitating the birthing process to maintaining optimal intra-abdominal pressure. These important muscles also act as a "sump pump." Their rhythmical pumping is coordinated with the respiratory diaphragm, helping circulate blood and lymph so they don't congest in our pelvic region. Yes, not only our ankles but also our pelvic basin can become swollen if we sit too long. Any damage to one of the muscle layers will impact not just the area surrounding the damage, but also our overall health and lifestyle. Hence, it's important to understand the specifics of the three layers. Let's take a look.

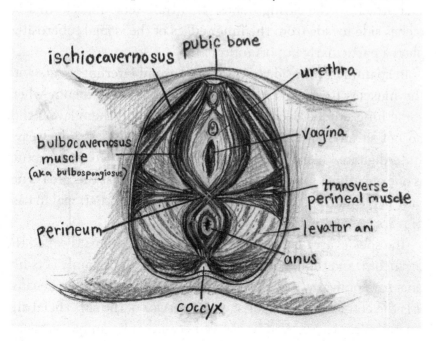

**Layer One:** The most superficial muscles of the pelvic floor are the bulbocavernosus, ishiocavernosus, superficial transverse perineal, and the external anal sphincter muscles. The bulbocavernosus and anal sphincter come together elegantly to give us a figure eight shape (or an infinity sign if you prefer) attaching in the front to the pubic bone and surrounding the urethral and vaginal openings. In doing so, these muscles create the area between vagina and anus, called the perineum, and from there circle back around the anal sphincter. (Sphincters are the ring-shaped muscles we find throughout the body that have the purpose of opening and closing; there are two sphincters in the pelvis, the urethral and the anal.)

**Layer Two:** The second layer consists of a group of muscles that can be thought of as a diaphragm. This is sometimes referred to as the urogenital diaphragm, or deep perineal pouch, and consists of a dense sheet of fascia along with the external urethral sphincter, the compressor urethrae, the sphincter urethrovaginalis (women only), and the deep transverse perineal muscles. The second layer has only one muscle that is transverse, the rest are related to our urinary function and all are nestled in the same fascial membrane. Take particular note in the illustration of the bands of muscles that attach to the sitting bones. This transverse muscle that attaches side to side from the inner edges of the ischial tuberosities plays a particularly important role.

In spanning from side to side, this second layer intersects with the muscles from layer one at the area of the perineum where something unique occurs. Even though we call them layers they do not sit atop each other. Rather the muscle fibers interweave, "interdigitate," like a piece of woven fabric. This woven structure is one of nature's ingenious tricks to make sure that this area is not only particularly strong but that it also remains functional in case of tears (as commonly occur during childbirth).

The special area between the genitals and the anus is called the perineum, and though not officially a muscle, it certainly acts like one. Anatomically, it is also known as the central tendon because it is the connecting area for several muscles of the superficial and intermediate layers. And no doubt because of its unique location, it is also known by many other names as well. Yoga teacher Mary Paffard calls it "the Gateway to the Earth." In yoga philosophy it is the location of the root chakra. In seedier parts of town, the name is a little less regal: it's known as the "taint." Some hold that this moniker is most likely derived from a combination of "it" and "ain't"—it ain't vagina and it ain't anus. However, it is a place where many important structures meet up.

Although only about an inch in diameter (average for the female body), the perineum is nonetheless at the center of a lot of different practices and processes. In the yoga world, for example, it's where *mula bandha* occurs. It has been massaged for pleasure and birthing. It has been torn, cut, and stretched beyond what we think is possible. It's the meeting place of all things clean and dirty, a beginning and an end and a separation between the apertures of pleasure and poo. The perineum is also the true center of the bottom of the torso, the middle of the infinity sign that makes up our outermost layer of muscle. Energetically, it is the place that connects the arches of the feet and the inner legs to the pelvis.[2]

**Layer Three:** The deepest and largest of the pelvic floor muscles is the levator ani, a Latin name that translates as "anus lifter." As desirable as this function is, the levator ani does a lot more than that. Attached to each side of the lesser pelvis, it consists of a broad and thin muscle group that's formed by three muscles (the puborecta-

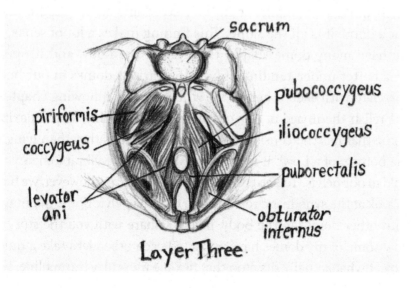

Layer Three

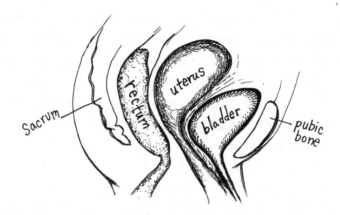

lis, the pubococcygeus, and the iliococcygeus). They surround the various structures that pass through this layer and support the viscera, the internal organs. Together with the coccygeus muscle, they make for the greater part of the pelvic floor.

Until recently, the levator ani has been completely misunderstood, or maybe I should say misrepresented. Even a cursory Internet search yields hundreds of images—all of which are *wrong*. They show the muscle shaped like a bowl or a hammock. The reason for this depiction is simple: that's what it looks like in cadavers. In the mid-90s, however, a study came out observing the levator ani in a living body, looking at it in real time and in full action.[3] What they saw was enlightening: far from sagging like a hammock, the pelvic floor appeared to actually have a slight dome to it—not as pronounced as the respiratory diaphragm (and definitely quite a bit smaller than the Astrodome or the Superdome), but a dome it is all the same. This finding makes a lot of sense, as we have many dome shapes throughout the body, and it opens up a better understanding of how the various domes in our body correlate with each other (as we will see in the following chapter).

I relish the image of our organs lightly bouncing atop a flexible dome that has the consistency of a trampoline, rather than lying at the bottom of a bowl. It is a radiant image of the vibrant energy we hold in our pelvis. To better understand this energy, however, we have to look at the synergistic relationship that the pelvic dome maintains with other domes in the body. Before I share with you the story of how some of my domes have impacted each other, let's take a quick look at what actually sits atop that flexible muscular trampoline.

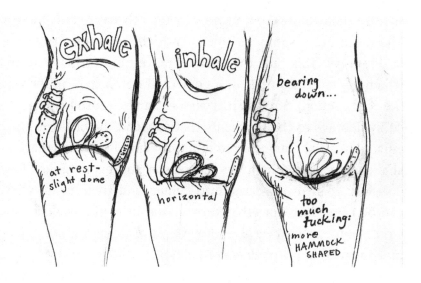

## Organs

The holy trinity of pelvic organs in the female body is (from back to front): the rectum, the uterus and the bladder. When each is in its optimal position, these three organs are constantly negotiating and renegotiating their space. The bladder fills and empties, the uterus swells and shrinks, and the rectum . . . well, we know what makes the rectum shift shape. All three lean against and support one another, and together they support the organs above them.

Allow me to introduce the bladder by way of a pungent idiom: A lively person can be described as full of "piss and vinegar." The history of this phrase appears to be a play on "vim and vigor" but implies devilish or mischievous behavior as well. And mischievous the bladder is. How else to explain all those incessant messages we receive that the bladder is full, only to find, once over the ceramic bowl, that there are just a few drops in there. Or worse, the bladder doesn't tell you it is full and you find out only because your drawers are suddenly wet. Or what about all the women who come to see me telling me they feel like they have a bladder infection but test results continue to come back negative? Let's take a look at how it works.

Think of the bladder as a balloon. As we take in liquid, the balloon begins to inflate, and the more it inflates, the more it leans onto the uterus. When we empty it, the bladder deflates and thus makes more space for the uterus. As the bladder gets fuller, pressure on the urethral sphincters, of which there are two, increases. The involuntary sphincter opens and lets you know it is time to find a potty. This puts the voluntary urethral sphincter to work, which hopefully is under your control (if not, help is on the way in the yoga section). Some urinary issues can be caused or exacerbated by damage to the ligaments that suspend the bladder. The ligaments can rip, tear, or stretch out, making bladder management challenging. This might be the reason the expressions "feeling pissy" or "pissed off" came into being. And some urinary issues can be caused or exacerbated by giving in to the bladder's every whim. Sometimes if we give into every urge to pee, we can create a misinformed brain/bladder connection.

> The uterus grows. The uterus retreats. It is not unlike the heart, a large, powerful muscle that swells, shrinks, twitches, and bebops. Oscillations and deep rhythms are the source of life, the principle of life; even cells work through pulsatile mechanisms. If we respond to music viscerally, it is because our viscera are the original percussionists, and the heart and the uterus are among the most perceptible of our natural pacemakers.
>
> —Natalie Angier, *Woman*

Directly behind the bladder sits the womb, also known as the uterus. It is the crown jewel, the keystone of a woman's body, the source of her creative force. She sits in the middle of all things arriving and departing. So strong is her energy that even if she is surgically removed, the creative force she carries still remains.

The womb has a shape similar to that of the heart, and indeed she is closely allied with many vital emotions. She signals a girl's passage to womanhood. She is intimately connected to the natural world, listening to its heartbeat, filling and emptying in rhythm with the phases of the moon. She is connected to the joy and passion of sexual desire and the bliss of finding out you are pregnant. She also endures the heartbreak of unwanted pregnancy and the tragic loss of miscarriage. The womb is the place where everyone starts, develops, and arrives from as a new human being entering the world.

Now you might think that the uterus, so crucial to the perpetuation of humankind, so rich in symbolic associations, would have a regal neighbor right behind her. Well let this be a "shout out" for rectum appreciation. Everyone thinks the rectum is full of shit and, well, the truth is that it often is. But that should be so only for short periods of time. Ideally, the rectum releases its contents at regular and predictable intervals. Furthermore, it is not only gross, but seems grossly unfair to our rectum that this natural process of elimination has been adopted as a metaphor for not telling the truth. The storing and dispensing of poop is an extremely important function, and, in my humble opinion, the rectum is its unsung hero. (However, people tend to underappreciate the rectum until they have experienced serious constipation.)

As the end of the line for the digestive tract, the rectum's work is facilitated through two sphincters, an internal one and an external one. When the rectum is full, the internal one opens, signaling to its owner that it's time to dispense. At this point said owner can only hope that one, the external one is at her service, and two, she is close to a bathroom.

Because the anal sphincters open and close every day (presumably), and are full of nerve endings, they tend to be the one area of the pelvic floor that we can most easily sense and become aware of. So sensitive are the anal sphincters that they are able to discriminate between solid, gas, and liquid. This sensitivity is no small thing, as an awareness of the many sensations in the pelvic area is critical to effectively diagnosing and overcoming troublesome conditions. In this sense, the rectum and anal sphincters are not only heroes but also role models.

Last but not least, we should not forget the one organ that surrounds our entire pelvis, as well as the rest of our body, this huge piece of breathable plastic wrap that all of us are enveloped in, the boundary between us and the world: our skin. Without it, we would literally be all over the place. It shields our inside from the outside (think extreme temperatures, chemicals, and such), produces essential proteins and vitamins, and retains what needs to be retained (for example, water). The skin is truly a masterpiece of nature's ingenuity, a living organism that completely renews itself about every 35 days—an amazing feat considering that every square inch of it has about 19 million cells.

The skin, threaded with thousands of nerve endings, tells us what we are and are not, and the skin of the vulva (the external female genitals) is particularly sensitive. The clitoris alone has about 8,000 nerve endings (which, by the way, is double the number in a

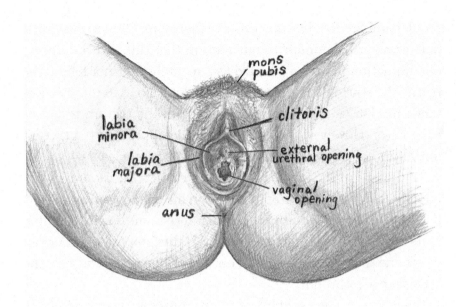

man's penis). The vulva is usually about the same color or a little darker than the rest of your skin. The inside of your vagina is more pink, close to the color of the inside of your mouth.

The shape and size of a woman's vulva can vary greatly. If you are curious about the wide range of different looks, I recommend you visit the art project "Wall of Vagina" by Jamie McCartney. Although I wish the artist would rename the project Wall of Vulva, the plaster molds of over 600 women aged 14 to 90 offer a fascinating view into what other women look like "down there." In a locker room men can always sneak a peek at each other and do a quick comparison. Women, on the other hand, can often see no more than a triangle-shaped fur patch a few inches below the navel—unless, of course, these other women have been graced by the topiary work of a Brazilian wax sculptress, in which case they may be sporting something more like a racing stripe. Or they've taken things to yet another extreme: the latest craze in pubic hair styling is the prepubescent look commonly known in waxing circles as "the Barbie."

~

This introduces another topic worthy of mention in our exploration of Pelvlandia; the topic of pubic hair and its role in keeping us healthy. As much as the clean and mean look of removing all hair is currently *en vogue*, it is important to know that it also carries a number of health risks. Shaving or waxing off all of your pubic hair leaves behind micro tears, which in turn can cause skin irritation, infections, and injuries. Pubic hair also provides a natural cushion against friction, and without this cushion we are not only more susceptible to bacteria and other unwanted pathogens, we are also at a higher risk of contracting genital warts. Although pubic hair doesn't completely prevent infection, it helps avoid skin on skin contact with someone who may already have the malady.

A last consideration concerning the value of pubic hair is that, as we sweat, our bodies produce sexual secretions known as pheromones. These pheromones are retained in our pubic hair and are a good part of what attracts our partners to us. By cutting it off, we may be cutting off a major source of sexual attraction. Sandra Cisernos writes:

> Once, watching a porn film, I saw a sight that terrified me. It was the film star's *panocha*—a tidy, elliptical opening, pink and shiny like a rabbit's ear. To make matters worse, it was shaved and looked especially childlike and unsexual. I think what startled me most was the realization that my own sex has no resemblance to this woman's. My sex, dark as an orchid, rubbery and blue-purple as *pulpo*, an octopus, does not look nice and tidy, but otherworldly. I do not have little rosette nipples. My nipples are big and brown, like the Mexican coins of my childhood.
>
> When I see *La Virgen de Guadalupe* I want to lift her dress as I did my dolls' and look to see if she comes with *chones* (underwear), and does her *panocha* look like mine, and does she have dark nipples too? Yes, I am certain she does. She is not neuter like Barbie. She gave birth. She has a womb. Blessed art thou and blessed is the fruit of thy womb . . . blessed art thou, Lupe, and therefore, blessed am I.[4]

So in regards to pubic hair, let us support a woman's right to choose. Whether you sport "bushiness," trim or wax in preparation for bathing suit weather, or model yourself after Barbie by removing all of it, let's be proud of our bodies and embrace the choice of informed fur management.

### Dome Dialogues

You have probably heard of the butterfly effect, which posits that an action as small as the gentle flap of a butterfly's wing may cause something as big and powerful as a tornado. The basic idea is one that we are all familiar with: changing the initial conditions in any given system can create effects that reverberate and magnify throughout that system, leading to potentially unpredictable and dramatic outcomes.

Fortunately, the mechanics of our body systems tend to be a little more predictable than global weather patterns, but the concept is as relevant: any change in conditions in one area of the body has effects in another, so it's necessary to understand how muscles in different parts of the body speak with each other and the mechanics that connect them. Let me tell you a story that illustrates the interconnections of my body. I call it "Can Someone Please Get All These Men Out of My Mouth?"

When I was an infant, my mother's male physician told her that breastfeeding was no longer necessary, and that baby formula was a perfect food. So my first "taste" of the world came through the rubber nipple of a plastic bottle filled with a substance concocted by scientists and business people for infants. The benefits of breastfeeding for the infant's immune system and oral cavity development is well documented: Bottle-fed babies have a narrowed upper palate, and that can contribute to overcrowding of teeth and a need for orthodontics.[5] Then, add to a narrow palate many years of highly processed soft food diet, and by age 12 my teeth were very crooked and full of mercury fillings. The family dentist had some simple advice. My mouth was "just too small for this number of teeth," he said. He sent me to his buddy down the street, the orthodontist, whose "easy solution" was to remove four bicuspids along with my wisdom teeth, wrap each tooth with a metal sleeve, thread two wires through the sleeves, hook up rubber bands connecting top to bottom, and tighten the wires and the bands every month. "She'll have a beautiful smile in just four years!" he assured us.

I resisted, I protested, I cried—to no avail. "You will thank me some day," my unwavering and well-intentioned father said.

The day my braces came off four years later, I stood in front of the mirror and wept. My mouth and smile seemed *so* very small. It took weeks before I stopped thinking how ugly my smile was, although by then I had fully mastered the art of smiling without showing teeth. Following the removal of all that metal, the orthodontist instructed me to wear retainers every night to keep my small, tight smile . . . well . . . small and tight. Now I finally had some control over what was going into my mouth. In a willful act of defiance, I refused to wear the retainers. It was my only way to say "Enough!" to all the men that had entered my mouth uninvited. My father had been mistaken. I have never felt the need to thank him.

The procedure shrank my palate and jaw and narrowed my face.[6] The roof of the mouth ideally should be a wide and low dome shape. My palate looked like the vaulted ceiling of a cathedral, tall and narrow. But more to the point, I noticed that these dental procedures seemed to adversely and dramatically impact other systems in my body. While the procedures I endured were hardly akin to the gentle flap of the beautiful creature's wing, the large-scale consequences were comparable to a tornado.

A wide dome in the mouth is preferable to a narrow dome. There's more room for your teeth and nasal passages, and a nice, wide space for the tongue to rest in. The roof of the mouth is just one of the domes in our body. We have domes from bottom to top: the arches of the feet, the pelvic floor, the respiratory diaphragm, the cervical diaphragm, the palate, and the cranial diaphragm. Ideally, in a healthy body, these domes or diaphragms move in unison. Our breath moves the respiratory diaphragm, whose movement affects all the other domes in the chain. In theory, every dome widens on inhalation and narrows on exhalation, creating a fluid, full range of motion dialogue. Conversely, if there is damage

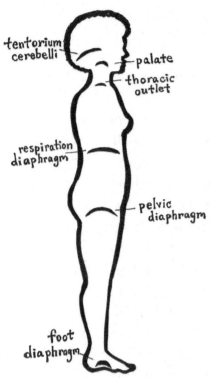

tentorium
cerebelli

palate

thoracic
outlet

respiration
diaphragm

pelvic
diaphragm

foot
diaphragm

or trauma to any one dome, the range of motion of the other domes may be compromised.

Here's where things get really interesting. The roof of the mouth, the hinge of the jaw, and the root of the tongue are all connected to the pelvic dome, both energetically and through fascia. Hence, if you grind your teeth at night, this can be an indication of excess tension in your pelvic muscles. A bound mouth can contribute to a bound pelvis and vice versa.

In my case, the braces and dental work that I had for a prolonged period of time led to movement restrictions in nearby and maybe far away muscles and tissues. Much of my worst dental trauma took place on my upper right side, with pain reflecting up the right side of my skull to the crown. When I was diagnosed with hypertonic pelvic floor, my right side was noticeably worse, and it took me significantly longer to ease tensions there. Where and when did this start? How did it all happen? Are they interconnected? Those questions may be as pointless as parents asking the same of their quibbling children. I'll never know for certain whether the point of origin was the mouth or the pelvis, but it doesn't matter that much. What matters is that all the domes of the body talk to each other; they communicate, they move and dance together, and when one dome is happy, the others respond in kind.

Let's take a closer look at the mechanics of the two muscle systems that have an immediate impact on the pelvis: diaphragmatic breathing and the pelvic floor muscles.

### Breathing and the Pelvic Floor Muscles

The average person takes in about 10 breaths per minute, equaling a total of more than 17,000 a day (the normal range extends to about 20,000).[7] You might think we would have some familiarity with an action we perform so frequently, but the opposite is actually true. For most of us, the breath is such a consistent, habitual, and "normal" part of everyday existence that we don't even notice it, even when we are breathing in a sub-optimal way. Respiratory action doesn't require our attention, as it happens automatically, with or without our conscious control. Ventilatory patterns (speed and coordination of inhalation and exhalation) are controlled by the autonomic nervous system, the contractions and expansions of the diaphragm, the chief muscle we use for breathing, are primarily involuntary.

Yet just as we can influence our heart rate by calming ourselves (e.g., taking a deep breath), we can consciously control a great number of processes that directly influence our breathing. And as we will see, we can actually improve our pelvic floor health by becoming more aware of our breathing.

Our lungs are spongy and made up primarily of vessels and tubes (think air ducts). The air ducts feed into the alveoli, small cup-shaped sacks that protrude from the air ducts (each lung has a whopping 300 million). Their main function is the exchange of oxygen and carbon dioxide. The respiratory muscles get air into and out of the lungs, while the heart works together with the lungs to provide our cells with oxygen.

Our lungs sit in the thoracic cavity and rest on the respiratory diaphragm, a large dome-shaped muscle that connects to the lower inner frame of the ribcage. I remember the moment when I first saw a diaphragm in the cadaver lab. The beauty of its translucent shimmering dome-like structure struck me, its fibers glistening from the center toward the outer edges of the body. It's shaped like a vault with the diaphragmatic fibers majestically arching out to the sides and down from the central tendon.

The diaphragm is responsible for the bulk of the respiratory work. When the lungs fill with air on an inhalation, a whole lot of things start happening. For one, the diaphragm moves down by flattening its dome-like structure and in the process it "pushes" the organs below it. With each breath, the diaphragm changes the shape of our organs. But as the diaphragm moves down, it also allows the lungs and the ribs to expand in what is known as "circum-

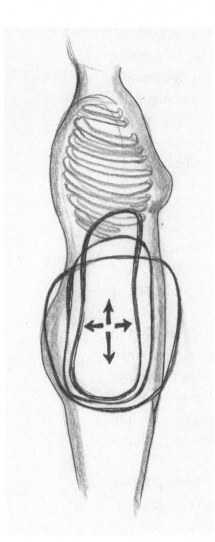

ferential" breathing. In circumferential breathing, the volume in the chest, belly, back, and ribs increases, thus expanding the whole torso. At the same time, our secondary breathing muscles, the intercostals (the muscles between the ribs and the abdominal muscles), are held in a gentle state of contraction, thus keeping the chest inflated. When we exhale, the transverse abdominal muscle (TVA) starts contracting, thereby increasing the pressure in the abdomen. When we exhale consciously, we can feel the TVA cinching like the strings of a corset.

Note in the illustration how the inhale expands the entire torso.

All of these processes have an immediate impact on the pelvic region. A healthy pelvic floor lifts in response to the TVA contracting and aids the TVA in exhalation while stabilizing the organs. The respiratory and the pelvic systems are intimately connected. Ideally, their movements are synced with each other. When the pelvic and respiratory systems are out of sync, like in reverse breathing, the effect on your health can be negative. Considering that we breathe between 17,000 and 20,000 times a day, our pelvic health depends on good breathing.

Now that we have a better idea of how our breath works with the pelvic floor, let's look at the muscle mechanics of the pelvic floor. Unlike the respiratory diaphragm, the muscles of the pelvic floor are voluntary. Generally speaking, the job of voluntary muscles is to move bones toward one another in response to conscious intent. For example, if my arm is hanging by my side and I want to bring food to my mouth, my biceps (upper inner arm muscle) has to contract and my triceps (upper outer arm muscle) has to lengthen. To bring the arm back down, the process is reversed, biceps lengthens, triceps contracts.

In the pelvic floor, our muscles can shorten into what is called a "concentric" contraction (think engaging the muscles to hold back pee or gas). They can also lengthen into what is called an "eccentric" contraction (think birthing a baby vaginally, or having your morning bowel movement). Both are vital for daily living. Also critical is the relaxation phase. A healthy muscle—be it our biceps, hamstrings, diaphragm, or any of the pelvic muscles—must relax fully after any contraction. Later on we'll get more into what can happen if this relaxing phase is impaired.

An oversimplified but easy and useful way to think about our pelvic floor muscles is in terms of their distinct front-to-back connections (pubic bone to tail) and some side-to-side connections (sit bone to sit bone). Thinking this way will help when we start finding and moving our own pelvic floors. There are many different ways of visualizing how to do it. For example, when the front-to-back muscles contract, the tailbone and the pubic bone move closer to one another (think tail tucking). When we tilt the pelvis anteriorly (remember anterior movement is sticking the tail out) so that we can lift and wag our tail, the muscles that run front to back are lengthening. The second layer, the urogenital diaphragm and deep transverse perineal muscle, run from side to side. Visualize this layer that attaches from sit bone to sit bone, so that when the transverse abdominal muscles engage, the sitting bones move toward each other. When we externally rotate the thighs, the sitting bones move toward one another, and the second layer contracts (shortens). When we rotate the femur bones internally, the sit bones widen, stretching the second layer.

So how does all this relate to our individual bodies? Just as everyone usually has one leg that's stronger and one that is more flexible, we have asymmetries in our pelvic floor. One side of our pelvic floor may be "smarter" than the other. Quite often, the less intelligent side is the culprit when it comes to our pelvic floor issues. Later, in the "Smart Ass, Dumb Ass" section (page 77), I'll talk more about this and how it relates to the gluteus muscles.

I had already traveled a long way on my pelvic journey before I discovered that my right side was a lot tighter than my left side

### Paradoxical Breathing

Paradoxical breathing, sometimes called reverse breathing, is when you pull the abdominal muscles in on the inhale, which activates the pelvic floor to lift. It may happen consciously or unconsciously. This habitual breathing pattern prevents the diaphragm and the pelvic floor muscles from descending.

Healthy relaxed breathing begins with a soft, wide inhale that expands the abdominal and pelvic floor muscles. It is easiest when lying down. The belly widens on the inhale and deflates on the exhale. Many of the women I meet in my workshops are reverse breathers, especially the hypertonic ones. This can be a reaction to trauma that becomes a habit.

Breaking this pattern and practicing deep abdominal breathing, or what I like to call whole-body breathing, has vastly improved my pelvic floor symptoms and those of my students. One study has shown that better breathing can even help with fecal urgency and incontinence.*

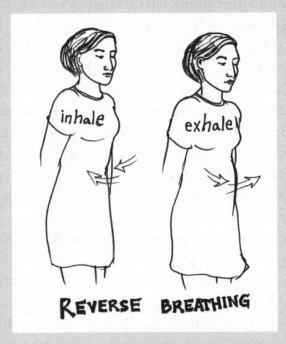

*Lynn M. Bartlett, Kathry L. Sloots, Madeleine J. Nowak, Yik-Hong Ho. Impact of relaxation breathing on the internal anal sphincter in patients with faecal incontinence. *Aust N Z Continence J.* 2012;18(2):38. connection.ebscohost.com/c/articles/82896609/impact-relaxation -breathing-internal-anal-sphincter-patients-faecal-incontinence, accessed June 13, 2017.

(although initially both sides were so tight I didn't notice the difference). Keep in mind that all combinations occur: We can be too loose or too tight on both sides; or we may be too stretched out on one, and simultaneously too tight on the other; or we may have one side that's relatively normal and healthy, but the other is not quite right. The only way for us to figure out what's what is through careful self-examination. The following section introduces a few exercises and techniques that will allow the curious explorer to set foot in the undiscovered country of Pelvlandia.

## Meet and Greet

### *Exploring through Breath, Touch, and Observation*

> If I hold a twenty pound weight, I cannot detect a fly landing on it because the least detectable difference in the stimulus is half a pound. On the other hand, if I hold a feather, a fly landing on it makes a great difference. Obviously then, in order to be able to tell the differences in exertion one must first reduce the exertion. Finer and finer performance is possible only if the sensitivity, that is, the ability to feel the difference is improved.
>
> —MOSHE FELDENKRAIS

The three best ways I have found for beginners to start exploring their own personal Pelvlandia are through breath awareness, palpation, and investigation of the effects. As we have discussed, some of our pelvic health conditions are related to our breathing. Our breath is easily accessible and hence an ideal starting point for exploration. The breath exercises below are chosen mainly for ease of use and for their diagnostic value. Later, we'll look at some of the more therapeutic ways of using our breath.

Another simple and powerful tool for exploration is touch. A simple massage can give us a lot of information about sensitivities, tender points, tensions, and more. I have included some guidelines appropriate to get us started for external and internal massage.

Finally, there is our posture, which can express our physical condition or conditioning and our emotional and psychological states. Just as with the breath, the more we can be mindful of posture, the more we can change it and improve the way we feel.

My hope is that you see these explorations not as arduous chores, but as fun and creative ways of getting to know yourself. I encourage you to play with these exercises, vary them in length, mix them with other exercises, practice them by yourself or with others—take any approach that fosters a natural and fun curiosity.

### Whole-Body Breathing

Lie down on the floor (or any other firm surface), support your head with a small pillow or folded towel, and place a rolled blanket or bolster under your knees.

Lay your hands on your upper chest between the collarbones and the breasts, and direct your attention to the movement of the breath. Set your intention as widening your breath so as to touch the inner side ribs. Observe your chest as the lungs fill. Pay close attention to the sensations in your left lung, then in your right lung as they inflate with each inhalation and deflate with the exhalation.

- Notice whether one side of your chest expands more easily than the other.
- Can you feel restrictions or tightness in one side of the chest more than in the other?

After a few minutes, slide your hands onto your belly beside the navel. Change your intention to start breathing deeply into the belly and pelvis. The movement of the breath will become less pronounced in the chest as you shift the focus of your attention to the sensations in the belly and lower back.

- Can you sense any differences side to side?
- How far down do you feel the body expand to receive the inhale? Is the belly inflating? Can you feel any movement created by the breath near the pubic bone?

Now expand your breath awareness to include the limbs, paying attention to the tips of your fingers and toes.

- Can you tell any difference in the effect on your body between the inhale and the exhale?

After a few minutes, let your awareness open up and feel your entire body breathing, gently rocking from the motions of inhaling and exhaling; feel all the different parts responding to one another, creating a myriad of sensation throughout the body.

- Does the movement of your breath flow smoothly or does it feel obstructed?

- Does the breath touch the body evenly or does it feel forced in some areas?

- Is it easier to sense the breath in one side of your body than the other?

If you have a hand mirror and a good light, get into a position where you can see the perineum while breathing deeply. You may see the area expand and contract with the breath. And while you have all the tools out and you are there any way, check the skin of your vulva. What are you looking for? Freckles, skin lesions, or ulcerations. It is common to have freckles on the vulva but if you see a suspicious one, please check with your doctor.[8]

### *Synchronizing Breath and Movement*

Lie on a firm surface, support your head, and bend your knees so that the soles of your feet rest evenly on the floor.

Place your fingertips on the pubic bone and start tilting your pelvis back and forth (anterior and posterior), tucking and un-tucking as in cat-cow yoga poses. As you bring your lower back into the floor, your tail goes toward the ceiling, which is a tuck; as you arch your lower back away from the floor, your tail moves away from the ceiling, which is an untuck.

Begin to synchronize the movement with your breath. Tuck on the exhale, untuck on the inhale. Repeat that for a minute or two until the synchronization feels smooth and organic.

Then begin to minimize your movements, making them small-er and smaller until you are no longer rocking the pelvis. You may notice that the pattern you just practiced is nothing but an exaggerated form of what is already happening: when we breathe correctly and deeply, the pelvis moves anteriorly on the inhale and posteriorly on the exhale.

**Notice:** If this breathing/moving exercise does not come naturally to you, or if you have a tendency toward the opposite (i.e., your pelvis moves posteriorly on the inhale and anteriorly on the exhale), you are what is called a "paradoxical breather" or a "reverse breather." This is a condition common to many of my students with pelvic health problems.

### Facilitated Side-to-Side Breath

Lie on a firm surface, support your head, and bend your knees so that the soles of your feet rest evenly on the floor. Place your fingertips on the right and the left side of your ilia (the fronts of the hip bones) and begin to gently push your right foot into the floor. You will notice that the right side of your pelvis is more anterior, and the left side is more posterior. Then reverse the action, and do the same with the left side. The movements are similar to those when we walk.

Note how the subtle motion impacts your breathing. When you push with the right foot and the pelvis goes anterior, you may find it easier to breathe deeply into the right side of the abdomen; opposite movement may facilitate breathing into the left side.

### External Massage

A little massage is an ideal way to develop greater awareness of this area.

In any seated position, lean onto your left buttock so that the right sitting bone is easily accessible (you can also do this lying on your side). Using either hand (whichever is more comfortable), find the tip of the right ischial tuberosity, a.k.a. sitting bone. Using the sitting bone as your landmark, begin to massage the muscles just on the medial side (inner edge of the sitting bone toward the vulva). Massage a little toward the front and a little toward the back, and see if there are any tender or tight spots in the corridor between your vulva and the bone. Take note of the density of the muscle around the bone. Is it firm, hard, squishy? What does the shape of the bone feel like? Continue for 1 full minute.

• Are you noticing any tenderness, sensitivity, or even pain?

• As your fingers glide over the sitting bone, what does the shape feel like and what is the density of the muscle?

• Does the area have any "give"? Is it firm or does it feel tense?

Now sit back on both sitting bones and observe the difference between the right and the left sides.

• Has anything changed as a result of releasing muscular tension on one side?

• Does the right sitting bone feel lower on the seat? Is there a sense of more space around the bone?

Now take a few deep breaths and shift your attention to the breathing sensations.

• Does the right side of your body feel more spacious as you inhale? Repeat on the left side and notice any differences.

### Internal Massage

Healthy pelvic muscles should be pain-free—period. We should not have pain with urination, defecation, sex, sports, or at rest. Likewise, gentle to moderate internal vaginal massage should be pain-free in healthy women. That said, tension is commonly held in this area, so if you find a painful area, try to breathe into it and see if it relaxes over a minute or so. We all hold tension at certain times and it might just let go. But sometimes the muscle tension doesn't let go so easily and you may need a little extra help. I strongly encourage you to seek out a physical therapist (P.T.) or occupational therapist (O.T.) with a pelvic floor specialty who is qualified to work internally.

With regard to self-massage, first make sure you are in a place where you feel safe and have some privacy. You can perform the massage lying down, seated on the edge of a chair on a towel, or standing with one leg up on the edge of a chair. Make sure to wash your hands before starting (you can also use medical-grade gloves) and that you don't have ragged fingernails. Imagine the circular opening of the vagina as having the face of a clock so that the front of your body is the noon position; with the clitoris and the urethral sphincter marking 12 o'clock, your left inner thigh is 3 o'clock, to the right is 9 o'clock, and the perineum or the back of your body is 6 o'clock. Do not massage near the top 10 to 2 positions without professional guidance as you may irritate the urethral opening.

Using a lubricant (I like coconut oil or Vital V Wild Yam Salve from MoonMaid Botanicals), gently insert your thumb or a vaginal dilator at a slight angle into the vaginal opening, and massage the muscles from about 2 o'clock until about 10 o'clock.[9] (I mean the *position* here; doing this for eight hours would be a problem.)

Now what is internal massage supposed to feel like? Here's a helpful analogy: If you completely relax one arm, you can push into your biceps without much resistance. When you bend your arm, you will feel the biceps firm up. Similarly, when you are consciously trying to relax your pelvic floor during the massage, the muscles should have some "give," as with the relaxed biceps. If you feel pain, tenderness, or hardness (some women have described it as feeling

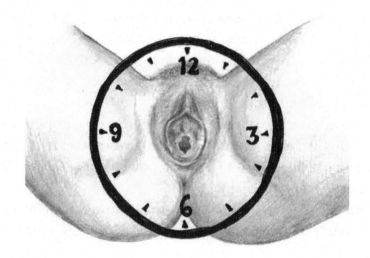

like a taut guitar string), this indicates there is too much tension in the muscles. Remember, we want muscles that have healthy tone, which means they can contract and soften appropriately.

It is crucial that you tune into your breath the whole time you are performing internal massage. Check the depth of your breath before you start, do regular breath checks while massaging and then again when you are done. The breath is your guide here. If you experience a shallow breath or find yourself holding your breath, back off or stop completely until you can return to deep breathing.

Note that if your muscles are particularly tight, you may not be able to get inside the vaginal opening. If that is the case, simply massage around the vaginal entrance and at the perineum. Over time, you will find that you can slowly make progress with vaginal entry, even if you have to use your pinky finger. If you have tightness or pain around the entrance of the vagina, try placing the finger on one spot and applying very gentle pressure. When you can do that while taking a deep breath, begin to move your finger in a small, circular movement. Another technique is to hold your thumb or index finger in place inside the vaginal opening and very gently tug on the muscle, holding it in a stretched position for a few breaths.

When you encounter a sensitive area, lessen any pressure until you can fully relax and breathe deeply, then slowly increase pressure. Visualize or draw an actual map of all the spots that are sensitive, cause pain, or feel "hardened." You can keep it simple—draw a clock face and note exactly where there are any tender points. For example, the most painful spot is at 3 o'clock, while 5 and 6 o'clock are sensitive.

You may want to pause between sides during internal massage and feel the effects on your breath and the rest of your body. For example, I notice that after massaging the right side of my pelvic floor, the tension in the right side of my neck eased and facilitated deeper breathing on that side.

Massage each side for 2 to 5 minutes. If you are within normal range or tend to be more on the lax side, there may be no pain or discomfort at all. In that case, push your thumb more to the right side and contract your pelvic floor; then repeat on the left. Gauge how well you were able to contract your muscles.

- How responsive are the muscles?
- Does one side respond better than the other?
- Could you hold your finger with your pelvic floor muscles?

If you still have your flashlight and hand mirror handy it is also important to make sure when you think you are engaging the pelvic floor that you really are. Some women think they are lifting their pelvic floor or doing a Kegel and in reality they are bearing down. This is not uncommon and so it is important to check that what you are feeling is actually what is happening.

If you are menstruating regularly, it is helpful to map your cycle and correlate it with this exercise. In my own cycle, I found that my pelvic floor muscles softened quite a bit a day or two before my period started. If you have a hypertonic pelvic floor, massaging and feeling the quality of your muscles before menstruation can give you some reference for what soft muscles feel like. Please note that some women who have bad menstrual pain can actually tighten more before their periods, possibly in anticipation of a painful period.

### Posture and Sitting

An important part of body awareness is becoming more conscious of your posture. Check your posture right now: What's the position of your pelvis as you are reading this? If you are sitting, is your tail deeply curled under you in the same fashion as a dog when it's scared? Are your sitting bones lined up next to each other, or is one forward and the other back? Are you actually on your sitting bones or are you on the gluteus muscles and tailbone? How aware are you of your posture, in general?

Many of us have developed a habit of sitting *behind* the *ischials* (sitz bones or sitting bones). When we do that, the bottom of our sacrum and the tailbone are pushed forward, leaving the organs unsupported. Another common habit is to sit in a chair with one leg crossed over the other. When we sit like this, we tuck our tails under and then cross one leg over. This posture restricts blood flow and creates an imbalance in the pelvic floor. This imbalance, if repeated often enough, will eventually show up in our bone structure, as bones react to the forces put on them by changing shape. Perhaps most egregious of all, this cross-legged position limits our ability to take a deep breath. Try it.

For many women, having to sit for long periods of time is a job hazard; it's unfortunate, but unavoidable. That makes it all the more important to develop better awareness of our sitting posture, because only by noticing it can we correct it, adjust it, and create new habits.

If you have to sit, sit on your sitting bones. In yoga class, when we are seated on the floor or blankets, we are often instructed to pull the flesh out from underneath our sitting bones. Please note that it is safer for the hamstrings, especially if you have a hamstring injury or are trying to avoid one, to grab the top part of the hamstring when adjusting the flesh of the buttocks back to allow yourself to come on to the sitting bones. I recommend that you do this anytime you are seated, whether in your chair at work or in your car. Basically, pull the flesh out from under you whenever you can do it without causing the people around you to think about public indecency. Adjusting our posture so that we are atop our sitting bones helps blood flow to the pelvic floor muscles and helps the spine line up in a neutral, healthy position. If you sit more toward the back of the sitting bones, you lose some of the lumbar curve; if you sit too far forward on the sitting bones, the spinal muscles harden and compression may occur in the lower back.

For most of us, the idea of a "neutral" pelvis, along with the front, back, and center of our sitting bones, is a very foreign concept. But once you develop the ability to discern the differences, you will start to notice your habits: Do you often fall back and flatten the lumbar curve? Do you tend to sit in front of your sitting bones and get lower back pain? The more awareness you develop about your sitting habits, the more readily you will be able to make the correct adjustments. Be vigilant about your seated posture and you may soon find that your pelvic floor already feels better, that you breathe more easily, and that life may just seem a little better.

### Standing

Many women stand with their pelvis and femurs hanging forward, which puts the pelvis in a posterior position, and with their hips thrown to one side. As an example, take the multitasking mother who has her baby perched on her hip while engaging in a task with her "free side." She is very likely to have a preferred side for holding the child, and a preferred side for doing other tasks, most likely based on her left- or right-handedness. She never switches those sides. Now remember, when the pelvis is posterior (tucked or retroverted) the pelvic floor muscles are shortening. When standing with the pelvis tilted this way, the body weight is hanging forward in the groin area. This has a whole lot of unintended consequences. For one, it can stress the ligaments in the front of the hip socket, which can contribute to hip pain. Also, in this position the pelvic organs are not supported by the pubic bone. This puts the burden of support on the ligaments that hold our organs and they may already be stretched out. The pelvic floor muscles may also already be overstretched and weak, or shortened and weak.

Ideally, we should stand with our weight distributed equally on both feet and keep our pelvis atop the legs. I highly recommend a standing desk, one that you can adjust throughout the day in order to stand, sit, and perch. Yes, that's right, perch. I learned about perching in *The Chair: Rethinking Culture, Body, and Design* by Galen Cranz, Ph.D., a professor of architecture at the College of Environmental Design at the University of California,

Berkeley. Perching is a cross between sitting and standing. Think of sitting on the edge of a high stool so that your legs are almost fully extended with the feet flat on the floor and you've got perching. A standing desk will take some time to get used to, especially because we've grown accustomed to sitting so much. Don't give up. It can take almost a year to get comfortable with sitting and standing correctly.

### *Proper Sitting in the Small Room*

Among all the emails I get from folks who have attended my workshops, the most effusive ones come from women who thank me for my "poop talk." Sitting improperly in a chair is not conducive to pelvic health. The same holds true for how we sit on the toilet. One of the problems with a standard toilet is that it encourages us to tuck our butt under, especially the oval-shaped toilet ring. This position forces the anal canal into a forward-facing position rather than a downward position, which makes it a lot more difficult for waste to get through and out of the intestinal tract and bowels.

If you have spent time around small children, you know that squatting to defecate comes naturally to them. It is the better way to "go" and, in fact, many people around the world relieve themselves in this position using squatting toilets.[10] But somehow we Westerners got it into our heads that the "squatting to poop" method could be improved upon, and we engineered the Western toilet. We should have kept our heads out of our butts. Squatting to poop naturally opens up the butt cheeks, puts the anal canal into the optimal position for release, and creates a natural downward pressure in the pelvis. If you suffer from a rectocele, hemorrhoids, or constipation, squatting to poop could change your life.[11] Please check with your healthcare practitioner about squatting if you have a prolapsed organ. Generally, squatting is not recommended with prolapse.

What exactly do I mean by squatting? Bearing in mind that the ring-shaped toilet seat is not built for folks to squat upon, I am

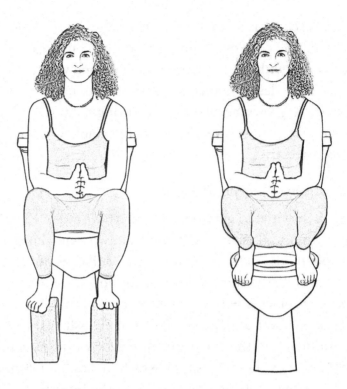

not necessarily advocating that you climb up onto it (although I do). Instead, you can assume a modified squatting position simply by using a footstool or setting up two yoga blocks for your feet at the base of the toilet. Raising your feet off the floor in this way approximates squatting pretty well.

We are very often creatures of habit. But that doesn't mean that habit and correct are always synonymous. Sometimes what we do habitually makes things worse. Examining, re-evaluating, and possibly experimenting with all our postures—seated, standing, and squatting—is a great way to develop better body awareness and take charge of ourselves. We can implement small changes that have major effects on our well-being.

### Beyond the Perineum

So far, we have taken a look at our bits, checked the skin of the vulva for suspicious looking freckles, sensed our breathing, and given ourselves an internal massage to see if there is pain or sensitivity. Hopefully at this point you have a sense of how happy or unhappy your pelvis is. Next, we'll do something that will require time and patience, but it's absolutely crucial if we want to understand—in our minds, in our bodies—what exactly our pelvic floor is and what it is not. We will attempt to move the different muscles of the pelvic floor in such a way that we can feel their differences. If we develop a nuanced sense of both their position and function, we can use this knowledge when working with the pelvic floor in yoga. By stretching and strengthening the pelvic floor, we can feel how the different yoga poses affect specific muscles.

~

Choose a comfortable seated pose, it doesn't matter which one as long as you keep the pelvis in neutral; that is, you should be on your sitting bones with the perineum parallel to the ground and the spine in its natural curves. Remember, no tail tucking. Sit with the crown of the head reaching skyward, and imagine your tail regally resting behind you.

Find a small, soft item and place it up against the perineum.[12] A yoga belt works well. Take the non-buckle side of the belt, and roll it up until it's about three-quarters of an inch in diameter; then place the belt such that it is comfortable and pushing up into your perineum. If you don't have a yoga belt handy, take a washcloth,

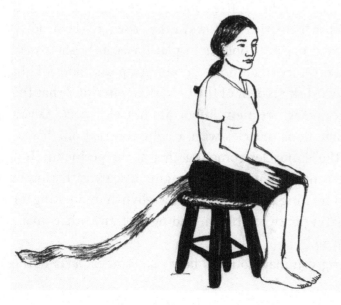

roll up one corner, and put it up against your perineum. I have also used toy balls with rubber strings attached to a soft rubber core (think of your item as a little baby bolster for your perineum). This exercise is designed to deepen your awareness of this small, specific place in your body.

With your item in place, breathe slowly and deeply and bring your attention to the perineum. Do you feel a difference in pressure against the item on the inhale and on the exhale? Can you describe what you feel? Ideally, you will notice a little more pressure against the item on the inhale and less on the exhale. This exercise can be really effective for waking up the perineum and can help you discriminate between some of the different sensations.

Don't worry if you are not able to feel a difference between the inhale and the exhale—that will come with practice. Now we are ready for our first active contraction of the pelvic floor, the lifting of the perineum. Remember, ideally the pelvic floor will lift on an exhale as part of good breathing. Now we will try a very small contraction of the perineal area by lifting up on the exhale and then letting go on the inhale. The operative word here is *small*. If we use too much force, larger muscles like the quadriceps and buttocks will get involved, making it harder to sense what we want to feel. When it comes to learning how to engage the pelvic floor, less is more. As a general rule, use about 25% of your full strength when trying to lift the perineum toward the crown of the head.

Now, with your perineal bolster in place as you begin a new exhale, visualize the perineum area doming up and add a light contraction toward the crown of the head. Keep in mind that the perineum is the area where many important muscles meet. As you engage the pelvic floor muscles with a light contraction, visualize how all of these muscles come together at the perineum. If it helps, here are some visualizations: Imagine a scarf gathering in the middle and floating up and down, or a jellyfish undulating, or a flower alternating between bloom and bud, or any other image that works for you.

The first thing you may notice is how many other parts of the body are trying to get involved. The anal sphincter is usually the first to come to the party. If you have this level of awareness at the anal sphincter, nudge your awareness slightly forward so that the lift starts at the perineum and the sphincter then follows. You may notice a variety of sensations, such as the twitching of buttock muscles, the grinding of the jaw, or the hardening of the sides of the throat. When you learn a new movement in the body, be aware that many other parts of the body will try to help. Confusion about these kinds of exercise is common; it's a normal and healthy part of the learning process. Most of us have never examined this part of our bodies with such specificity, so be patient.

### *Squat Pose (*Malasana)

The perfect squatting position in which to poop is a yoga pose called *malasana. Malasana* is also ideal for exploring and finding the pelvic floor muscles. Please do a modification of *malasana,* lying on your back, if you have a prolapse.

From a mountain pose (*tadasana*) position, with feet hip distance apart, place a rolled blanket under your heels.[13] How big the roll should be depends entirely on how tight your muscles are. For most of us, when we squat, our heels come off the ground and our butts tuck under. The rolled blanket (or sticky mat or even a pair of high heels) has to be tall enough to support the heels and allow the pelvis to remain in a neutral position. If your pelvis is not in a neutral position, you need to adjust the height of your support (as if you have your highest stiletto heels on).

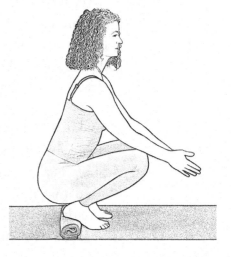

Once in the squat, fully bend your knees, so that your butt comes toward the back of the heels. Now that you are in *malasana*, begin to tune into feeling your inhale and exhale in the pelvis. This pose is one of the best to isolate your pelvic floor. With each exhale, visualize a circle drawn around the area of the perineum; visualize its central location and what the

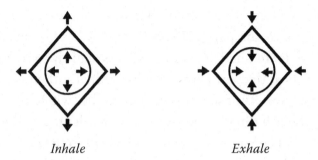

*Inhale*                    *Exhale*

In the above diagram, the four points of the diamond
shape represent the pubic bone, the tailbone, and
the two sitting bones. The circle represents the
perineum. When focusing on your breath, visualize
the pelvic diamond and perineum widening as you
inhale and narrowing as you exhale. Add in movement with the breath. On the inhale (cow pose), the
diamond widens, and on the exhale (cat pose), the
diamond narrows.

muscles look like, and then gently lift. As you lift, there is a slight
narrowing of the circle as it travels upward, toward the crown
of the head. As you inhale, let go and imagine the space of the
perineum widening. When we breathe in, the pelvic floor receives
the breath and the breathing diaphragm pushes the organs down.
As we exhale, the organs move back up in response to the breath.
If you know that you are hypertonic (tight pelvic floor), I would
recommend this pose be done passively, which means staying in
the pose for as long as your body allows, and taking deep "pelvic
floor–centric" breaths. This allows your pelvic floor muscles to
stretch passively with each inhale.

### Modified *Malasana*

If you find it challenging to stay in *malasana* for any length of
time, then try an alternative version. First, sit on a yoga block in
a squat position. Be sure to adjust the height of the block to make
sure that your pelvis is neutral and your tail is not curling under.

If you have knee issues, but still want to try the upright version, put a roll (a rolled yoga mat or a blanket) behind your knees. Sometimes this can reduce or alleviate pain in the knee. If that doesn't work, lie down and draw your knees halfway into your chest (if you draw them in too far, your tailbone will start tucking). Once you have found the appropriate *malasana* for you, pay attention to the breath as described above.

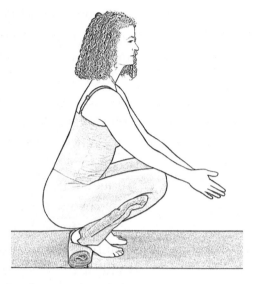

Generally speaking, the pelvic floor works hardest when you are sitting or standing, as that's when it bears the most weight. Hence, a great position to find and feel your pelvic floor is on your hands and knees as that shifts the weight of the organs to the front of the body. Similar to *malasana*, this position prevents the buttocks from getting overly involved. It's also most beneficial if there is a prolapsed organ. In this position, the organs no longer sit on the pelvic floor, but rest on the lower abdomen. Start with hands on the floor directly below the shoulders and knees directly below the hips.

Most of us have been in this kneeling position in the pose known as cat-cow, but I call it "tail play."

It's important to take a few moments to coordinate the movement with the breath. Inhale when the head and tail are going up (cow), and exhale when head and tail are moving down (cat). After a few rounds, stay on the hands and knees but bring the pelvis and head into a neutral position which is the halfway point between the two poses. Then, gently lift the pelvic floor on the exhale (many of my students find this the easiest position to access their perineum). If perineum access still seems elusive, slightly tuck your tail to move the pelvis posteriorly and try lifting the perineum. You will most likely notice that the feeling in the pelvic floor is slightly different this time, as the tip of the tail and the anal sphincter move more when the pelvis is tucked.

Then to contrast even more, go slightly past neutral into anterior tilt (tail up) and try to engage the perineum. When you do this, you will find that you are able to access the front of the pelvic floor much more easily. You may even feel the triangular shape of the urogenital diaphragm. How effectively you can activate the perineum indicates whether your pelvis is truly in a neutral position. If your pelvis is more tucked (posterior), you will be able to activate the back end of your pelvic floor more easily; if your pelvis is untucked (too anteriorly tilted) you will be able to squeeze the front of the pelvic floor more easily. But when your pelvis is in neutral, the perineum is most easily accessible to engage and lift.

### Delving Deeper

When you have a little more time and privacy, it helps to actually watch things happen. With a mirror in hand, find a position that allows you to take a look "down there." For some, propped up in bed with pillows behind the back is a good place. You can also sit on the edge of a chair, put the mirror on the floor and squat over it or put one leg up on a chair. Experiment and see what works best for you.

Take a few *deep* breaths. We want to think of the breath not just as something that fills our lungs or moves the diaphragm, but as something that moves our whole body. Breathing is a whole-body experience, and when we take deep breaths, we facilitate awareness of how it moves through us.

As you inhale and exhale, can you see any movement in the perineal area? If so, congratulations! You are a whole body breather. Note that this is not just your imagination, it is possible to *see* the breath moving the pelvic floor. Now with the mirror placed so you can see what happens, gently engage the anal sphincter.[14] You can see how it puckers and lifts up into the body, and how the perineum follows the sphincter. Then try the reverse order by changing your intention. Tell yourself you are going to start moving from the perineum and let the anus follow. Do you see a difference? Does it feel different? It might seem like a more gentle contraction.

As you do this, remember it's important to make sure that the perineum lifts and does not bulge down or out. The internal P.T.s I work with have told me that many women cannot feel the difference between contracting the pelvic floor and bearing down on it.

Next, try to squeeze only the walls of the vagina together and watch what happens. Then start the movement from the urethral sphincter. Ideally, both actions will allow you to see and feel more movement in the front of the pelvic floor.

Finally, attempt to lift only the right side of the perineum, and then only the left. Could you detect any visual or felt difference between the two intentions?

Like every other part of our body, the pelvic floor responds to gravity and positioning. It's fun to play around with this and try all the different movements while tucking the tailbone, and then try them again bringing the pelvis more into an untucked position (think tail up). What's crucial is to understand that what matters is where we initiate the movement. And it's crucial to know where our strengths and our weaknesses are.

A great pose to feel and maybe even see the pelvic floor stretch and contract is Goddess pose. Imagine the beautiful diamond shape that your pelvic floor creates between the tail, sitting bones, and pubic bone. At the very center of the diamond is the perineum. Come into Goddess pose (more detailed instructions are in the yoga section). As you bend your knees, stick your tail out and feel the pelvic diamond widen, and as you straighten the legs, imagine and feel your pelvic diamond narrowing.

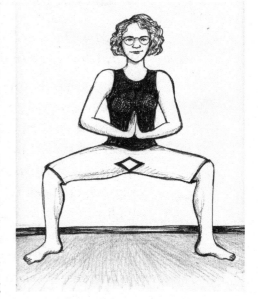

What if your perineum is damaged or frayed from tearing or being cut during childbirth? First, you or a pelvic floor physical therapist need to do some very gentle massage to bring blood flow into the area and hopefully break up any scar adhesions. Second, careful, mindful, and small movements of the pelvic floor can slowly bring your muscles back to health.

Cultivating this subtle awareness is the key to healing yourself. If you have a weak and a strong side and you do your contractions as if the sides were equal and even, you will likely end up making your stronger side even stronger, while your weaker side may stop engaging all together. Many women at my workshops tell me they had never noticed that one side wasn't engaging at all. This is one of the reasons Kegel exercises often don't work; women do them assuming their body responds symmetrically.

If we don't tune into what's going on in our pelvic floor, we won't be able to distinguish between movement patterns and ways in which the sides work differently from each other. When we can discriminate to the point that we can move and feel the front, the back, and the sides of the pelvic floor, it will be easy for us to tell the differences and work on them appropriately.

## What Your Mother Never Told You

### *Put More Junk in Your Trunk—*
### *Why Glutes Are Important for Pelvic Health*

Before yoga became my passion and occupation, I lived in the world of designers and architects in New York City. Whizzing up those tall skyscrapers, and feeling the buildings sway in the wind, I learned something important: stability is a good thing, but too much of it can turn into dangerous rigidity. Vertical structures like skyscrapers need to move; they need to be flexible to withstand high winds. Why exactly is that, I asked an architect friend. She explained that in a well-designed, stable structure, the different parts work together to balance out the pressure, whereas in a rigid structure a few elements bear all the stress, eventually weakening those elements.

The same principle applies to another vertical structure, our body. Ideally, our bodies are stable and flexible, but when the various parts and elements of our bodies are not optimally aligned, it shuts down some muscles and forces others to pick up the slack. And just as a structural imbalance in a building can't be fixed by putting tape and glue on it, we are not going to bring our bodies back into alignment with hair ties and lipstick.

Good engineering and asana have a lot in common. In architecture, we check blueprints and do stress tests on the material. In yoga, we look at our anatomy and try to figure out how to best strengthen our muscles. There is debate in yoga circles whether to work our glutes or let them just hang there, but to some extent this question confronts us with a false analogy. Remember, a tight muscle is not a strong muscle. This is an important distinction. We want to engage our glutes when needed but not clench our butts just for the heck of it.

My interest in butts (not a strictly anatomical term) grew out of necessity. I was doing bound angle pose (*baddha konasana*), actively pushing my heels together as instructed, when I noticed how asymmetrically my glutes were responding. The contrast was distinct. One gluteus was happily and fully engaged while the other felt like the dead butt zone. How could I have not noticed this before? Watching my students, I realized many of them had the same *smart ass, dumb ass* imbalance I did. This was something I needed to explore because I knew the impact our buttock muscles have on our pelvic floor.

Let's get to know this cheeky pair of orbs. There are three buttock muscles: gluteus maximus, gluteus medius, and gluteus minimus. Besides their obvious purpose of filling out your jeans so you

### The Pelvis

Richard Rosen

it's something like a bowl
but its bottom has a hole
and its rim's but halfway round
as a bowl it's quite unsound.

don't worry though it's not
made for liquids cold or hot
instead it works just fine
as a platform for our spine.

from here we've all been hatched
our legs are here attached
when weary on our feet
on it we take a seat.

from here we forward bend
male privates here suspend
and women's here are too
though they're hidden out of view.

though pelvis means "a bowl"
that's really not its goal—
it's where we store our gut
and a place to hang our butt.

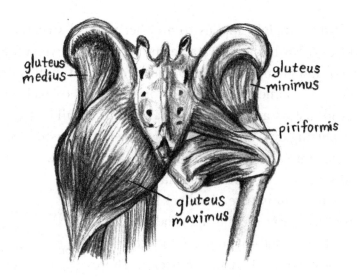

can ask your BFF if they flatter your posterior, one of their main functions is to stabilize your sacrum. They also balance and work against the pelvic floor. Two of the pelvic floor muscles attach to the anterior (front) side of the sacrum and pull it forward. Your buttocks muscles attach to the posterior side of the sacrum and make sure that the pelvic floor muscles don't pull the sacrum into too much of a posterior or tucked position. However, they won't be able to do that if you suffer from butt amnesia, that is, if your glutes have forgotten their job. The situation is no better if you are a perpetual butt clencher. In that instance, it may seem like the glutes are doing their job, but in reality, they are failing to balance the pull of the pelvic floor muscles and may even exacerbate pelvic floor tightness.

The gluteus muscles (commonly known as the butt) counterbalance the pelvic floor. If the pelvic floor muscles are short and weak, the gluteus muscles tend to be short and weak. If the glutes are overdeveloped, they can pull the sacrum too far back. Of the three butt muscles, the gluteus maximus, the largest and outermost one, gets the most hype. The maximus is responsible for hip extension (think the back leg when walking) and helps take the thighbone into external rotation. Then there is the gluteus medius; its main function is to stabilize the femur bone in the socket, particularly when we are weight-bearing (think of poses like tree pose [*vrksasana*]). The medius prevents us from falling over when we are walking. Finally, the gluteus minimus helps turn the femur inward and assists in flexion of the hip (think walking up stairs).

### Pelvic Inquiry

Let's look at mountain pose, *tadasana*. Bring your weight over the heels, so that the "eyeball" of the perineum is looking down and toward your heels. The quads should engage but not over-grip. The butt should have tone, but should not look and feel shrink-wrapped. The pelvis and lumbar spine should be in neutral, no tucking or untucking.

Place your hands on your glutes and see what happens when you begin to tuck your butt in this pose. If you tilt too much posteriorly (tail under), the butt shuts down and the hamstrings have to take over. This is how many of us live, in a permanent tuck. We tuck when sitting, we tuck when standing, and many of us have even managed to refine the art of tucking while walking.

The gluteus muscles have a lot of jobs and moving us across the earth is one of the more important ones. However, many of us don't engage our glutes when walking, thereby forcing other muscles to compensate. When we step forward (before the foot reaches the floor), our back leg buttock should be actively stabilizing us. When the front foot then hits the ground, our back leg buttock should fire to give us a push forward. But often that is not what happens. I spend a lot of time in airports where I watch how folks walk. Most people throw their front leg forward so that it is forced to catch the weight of the body, and then pull the hind leg after. This puts a lot of undue pressure on our hip sockets, and exacerbates the dead butt syndrome.

Many of us have short hip extensors (what we call the "groin area" in yoga) from too much sitting, and we have weak glutes, which are no longer pushing us forward. In a healthy body, the pelvic floor muscles and the gluteus maximus move synergistically in opposite directions when walking. The pelvic floor lifts up as we take a step, and the gluteus maximus engages to extend the leg backward. It is important that we maintain this synergy and practice engaging the buttocks in poses like goddess and chair pose (*utkatasana*).

Try this: Using a yoga block (or a stair step), place your right foot on the block as if about to step up, and place your left hand on your left buttock. Then step up, intentionally utilizing only the front leg (essentially dragging the back leg up). Do the left glutes contract at all? Then push off the left leg and foot to get you up the step and contrast that with what you just did. When you use your front leg only, you will notice that your back leg glute doesn't usually switch on; if you push off the back leg to step up, you should feel how the back leg glute is recruited.

The exact same principle is at work when we walk. Ask yourself: are you dragging or swinging your back leg forward, or are you pushing off of the back leg to walk? Try these three walks, first with shoes on, then barefoot:

1.  Walk across the room with your butt clenched.
2.  Walk across the room with your buttocks fully relaxed.
3.  Walk around the way you normally do, and see what your butt is up to.

What happened (besides your spouse questioning your odd behavior)? Do you have a pronounced tendency toward clenching or relaxing? What did you feel? Was glute recruitment equal on both sides?

Constant butt clenching can be an unconscious habit, or it can be a sign of hip or sacral misalignment. I used to be a "single butt clenchie," in that I would stand in line at the grocery store and for no known reason I would clench my right buttock. As I became more aware of the issue, I would catch myself doing it all the time. In yoga classes, I see a lot of butts that are either off-line or in perma-clench, yet there's little attention paid to the correct action of the glutes. Today, I consider myself a dedicated butt awareness advocate. If the muscles in our butts are not working properly, this often indicates that the front of the hip is really tight and short, which can in turn seriously compromise your ability to move. Non-working butts can also contribute to tight lumbar muscles, which may lead to, among other things, posture problems or low back pain.

Here are some evaluation poses and exercises for the buttocks that will hopefully give you new butt awareness in life and in your yoga poses.

Ideally, in poses with hip extension, the hamstrings and the glutes simultaneously engage to create the action. However, if the glutes are weak (common in modern society), the leg is raised either solely with the hamstrings or with the hamstrings first and the glutes second.

In the following poses, you will evaluate your own tendencies. And then you'll practice turning each set of buttocks on at the same time in symmetrical poses and doing a few extra repetitions on your weaker side in asymmetrical poses.

## "Smart Ass, Dumb Ass" Evaluation and Practice

The next four poses are evaluative and can also be stand-alone poses used for strengthening your buttocks (or your less-than-ideal buttock). I do believe there should be a different word for buttock singular. I suggest "butti," and then I could name this section "Return of the Butti."

### *Half Locust* (Ardha Shalabhasana)

In some yoga classes you might be told to internally rotate the legs before doing this pose. Although the leg shouldn't be externally rotated, I'm more interested in you using your gluteus maximus to lift the leg. This version of the pose is used to evaluate the tone of the gluteus maximus and establish the extent of left-right imbalances. The importance of this pose cannot be overstated. In addition to revealing left-right buttock imbalances, the pose mechanics are similar to those of proper walking.

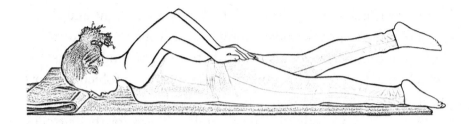

**How to Practice**

1. Lie on your belly with your forehead on a folded blanket.

2. Align the legs with the hips, tops of the feet on the floor. The distance between the legs is dictated by the distance between your hip sockets.

3. Place your arms beside your torso. Bend the elbows and place your fingertips in the center of the mid-buttock.

4. Keep both legs straight, pubic bone touching the floor and abdominal muscles lightly engaged. Lift your right leg.

5. Did you find any of the following: Did the buttock muscles engage (firm into the fingertips)? If not, the hamstrings were dominant. Did you feel any compression in your lower back? If so you might have lifted the leg too high or you were not able to get enough abdominal stability.

6. Repeat on the left side.

For some students, one or both buttocks are not engaged when doing this pose. Before moving on to the next pose, establish which buttock is less strong and has a harder time engaging. This is important.

Now, with more attention to details, try this:

To stabilize the lower back, lightly (which means don't forcefully suck your belly in) engage your abdomen away from the floor so that the pubic bone goes toward the floor.

1. Squeeze your right gluteus muscles particularly where the hamstring meets the gluteus. On an exhale, lift the right leg.

2. Do three to five lifts up and down, with the breath (exhale lift; inhale lower). Keep the leg lifted for 10–30 seconds.

3. Repeat on the left side.

If you find that one buttock isn't working as well as the other, do a few extra repetitions (10- to 30-second holds) and a few extra quick lifts on the weaker side.

### *Full Locust* (**Shalabhasana***)*

Now do the pose lifting both legs. If you found a left-right disparity, deliberately engage the sleepy buttock before lifting your legs.

**How to Practice**

1. Lie on your belly with your forehead on a folded blanket.

2. Place the fingertips in the middle of each buttock.

3. Engage your abdominals up from the floor.

4. Contract gluteus and hamstring muscles simultaneously.

5. On an exhale, lift both legs from the floor. Hold for 10–30 seconds. Be mindful that the legs stay straight.

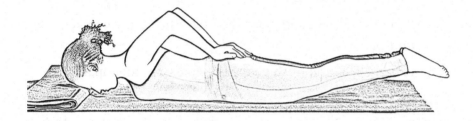

**Modifications**

If you still feel compression in your lower back, you can place a folded blanket under your belly between the navel and pubic bone.

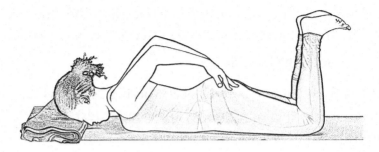

### Bow Variation (**Dhanurasana** *Variation*)

In this variation, the knees are wider than the hips in order to evaluate the gluteus medius and see if there is a left-right disparity. I learned this one from another pelvic floor goddess physical therapist in the Bay Area, Amy Selinger, P.T.

**How to Practice**

1. Lie on your belly with your forehead on a folded blanket.

2. Bend the knees and bring your shins perpendicular to the floor (at a 90° angle to your thighs). Keep the knees slightly wider than the hips.

3. Bring the back edges of the heels together so that the feet face away from each other.

4. Bend the elbows and place the fingertips in the center of the mid-buttock.

5. Flex the feet and push your heels together, toes apart.

6. Engage the abdomen.

7. Turn your gluteal muscles on. With your fingertips poking the buttocks, compare imbalances in firmness between left and right.

8. You are trying to turn on the glutes before the hamstrings, so if you notice an imbalance, push the heel on the lazy butt side into the heel of the harder-working side to try to activate the weak glute. Stay here for 10–30 seconds. Exhale to release.

### *Butt Ups (*Supta Padagushthasana *Variation)*

When practicing this variation you can feel the fibers of the gluteus maximus against the floor as feedback—or not, as the case may be. This pose helps evaluate disparity of strength in the left and right gluteus. This also has the added benefit of working the obliques (see Core Beliefs, page 87). I was taught this variation by an incredibly gifted movement teacher, Sarah Kotzamani.

**How to Practice**

1. Lie on your back with your legs extended on the floor.
2. Bring your arms by your sides. Bend the elbows so that the forearms are straight up, palms facing each other.
3. Raise the right leg perpendicular to the ground, flexing the foot so the sole faces the ceiling. If your hamstrings are tight, bend the right knee, so that the bottom of the foot still faces the ceiling. Keep the left leg straight.
4. Push the right elbow into the floor, firm the left gluteus, and lift the right leg to the ceiling. As you lift the right leg straight up (the leg will try to waver toward the midline; don't let it), allow the left leg to roll externally so that you're rolling from the inner to the outer butt. The right butt will come off the floor as you lift the right leg up.
5. Do 8–10 repetitions and repeat on the second side.

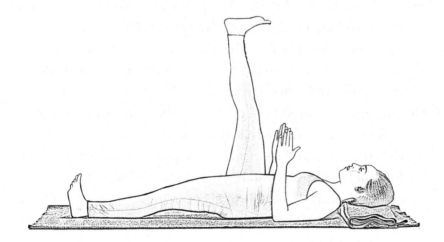

### Focused Actions

- Use the right elbow for leverage and directional guidance to lift the right leg, but try to get the left buttock to do the work. The right leg is lifted because of the work of the left buttock. If the left butt is weak, the push of the right elbow into the floor will try to compensate.

There are more poses with attention to the buttocks in the asana section. Please go to page 203 if you want to continue your "smart ass" practice.

## Speaking in Tongues

We hear it all the time: *It's all connected.*

As a yogini, I know this. And yet, when I experienced the mouth-pelvis connection for the first time it came as a complete surprise. Remember how Lizanne, my P.T., had released the right side of my pelvic floor through internal manipulation? Afterward, I noticed the chronic pain in the right side of my neck and jaw disappeared.

Over the course of several weeks, Lizanne worked to release my pelvic floor muscles even further, and I noticed a corresponding release and relaxation in my jaw, throat, and tongue. Having been a jaw clencher for years, I couldn't help but wonder—if releasing my pelvic floor has such an immediate impact on my mouth and jaw, could the reverse be true? Is it possible to improve pelvic floor health by working on the muscles of the mouth?

According to yoga philosophy, there is an important energy line that flows from the anus to the tip of the tongue. It is named after the Hindu goddess of knowledge, arts, music, and wisdom, Saraswati. Modern anatomy experts like Tom Myers have written about the "deep front line" of fascia that starts at the roots of the toes, goes through the pelvis and connects to the pelvic floor, then travels up the front of the spine to the root of the tongue. With all these connections, shouldn't we be able to effect change in either direction?

The physical practice of yoga has made me aware of how anxiety expresses itself in the body through tightening of the muscles. When we are frightened or upset, adrenaline (the fight or flight hormone) is released and immediately constricts the tissues in our body. Constricted muscles can make our vocal register rise, sometimes breaking, sometimes coming out in screeches. To find out more about what actually goes on, I contacted Cheryl Keller, a long-time voice teacher in Berkeley, CA. Cheryl explained that anxiety tightens our vocal cords and this causes the voice to ascend into the upper registers. Conversely, when our abdominal muscles relax, we can take in much deeper inhalations, which then allows us to access a much stronger voice.

Cheryl teaches whole-body singing. I teach what I like to call "whole-body breathing" because once I learned how to completely relax on an inhale, I could feel how much deeper my organs descended; how my whole body engaged; and how I was able to "belt it out."

Cheryl went on to explain that the larynx (think voice box/ vocal cords) attaches to the tongue and moves down with each inhale, allowing the jaw to relax and the tongue to become supple. "Do you think singing might help students with tight pelvic floors and, if so, why?" I asked her. She answered with an enthusiastic affirmative, explaining that "good singing is all about how big your inhale is. If the pelvic floor is constricted, you cannot get as big an inhale as you can with a supple pelvic floor. Practicing singing with conscious inhales, allowing the pelvic floor to descend, can help your pelvic floor *and* your voice."

In another field, midwives, doulas, and mothers who have given birth also know about the mouth-pelvis connection—if you want to relax the pelvic floor, relax the mouth and throat. Minneapolis-based midwife Gail Tully of Spinning Babies told me a wonderful story.

A young mother-to-be had been in labor for many hours, but her cervix had dilated only to 6 cm. A C-section seemed increasingly likely, but Gail asked for an hour to work with the mother and perform a protocol called "Dynamic Body Balancing," developed by chiropractor Carol Phillips.[15]

Gail and the mom-to-be undertook the protocol to its final stages in which the tongue unwinds and there is a release of the temporomandibular joint in the muscles of the mandible. In response, the woman's nasal bones released, and her sacrum flared out in response. The doctor returned with the paperwork to perform the C-section. Gail requested that they wait for three more contractions before having the woman sign the papers. "Just three more, and I think the mother will be ready to push," she told everyone. Indeed, on the fourth contraction, the woman gave birth vaginally by her own power . . . and maybe with a little help from releasing her tongue and mouth.

The tongue is often called the strongest muscle in the body. In Eastern medicine it is considered an internal organ that we have access to. We think of the tongue as a singular organ, but it's made up of many bands of muscle. It's crucial for chewing, swallowing, tasting, speaking, and, sometimes, other fun activities. The tongue is even at center stage in brain plasticity research. Researchers have found that stimulating the tongue can help some people recover mobility that they have lost from stroke, Multiple Sclerosis, and Parkinson's.[16] We should all get to know a little bit more about our tongues.

The root of the tongue is anchored in the hyoid bone, which is the only bone in the body that floats, meaning it is not attached to another bone. Instead, it is held in place by fascia. Shaped like a small horseshoe between your bottom jaw and your laryngeal prominence (Adam's apple, and yes, women have them), the hyoid serves as a flexible anchor to the tongue.

For proper function, it's vital that the tongue has full range of motion when necessary. But when it is at rest, it should relax completely. It tends to tense most when it lengthens from root to tip and is most at ease when it spreads from side to side like a soft wide carpet—wide enough that it touches the inner edges of the top teeth. Problems can arise when we don't know how to properly relax our tongue. But before trying to consciously relax and widen the tongue, it's helpful to become aware whether your tongue is tense.

The dome of the mouth is the floor of the nose, and it's commonly accepted that the natural resting place for the tongue is on the palate, just behind the front teeth. In this position, it supports the mouth dome, which in turn helps the nasal passages widen for better breathing. Some orthodontists assert that where we place our tongue contributes to our entire body posture. Michael Mew, D.M.D., clinical director of the London School of Facial Orthotropics, espouses that the whole tongue, in particular the first third of the tongue near the root, should adhere to the roof of the mouth as it supports your head and an upright position of your face.[17] Think of this as *tadasana* of the tongue.

Looking for additional insights, I went to see my friend and fellow yoga teacher Ann Dyer to talk "*tadasana* of the tongue." Ann has been involved with the art of chant and voice for over 35 years; she practices a type of yoga called *Naada Yoga*, or the yoga of sound. "In the Western approach to voice, you work a lot on your high notes," Ann explained. "The Indian approach is different; you work mostly on improving your low tones. And if you do that, your high tones will follow automatically." This approach is based on the insight that our breath and our ability to sing both come from the root chakra, which sits approximately at the perineum.

I asked her about the energy line that flows from the anus to the tip of the tongue. "Did you know that it was named after Saraswati?" I asked. "Makes perfect sense," she replied. "Saraswati, the goddess of music and learning, is an incarnation of the goddess Vak. Vak is said to be the goddess of word. And so when the universe was manifested, it was from a sound, and that sound was *om*."

Learning to work with our mouth, tongue, and jaw is not an exotic or tangential specialty; it can help us relax our entire body, foster healthier posture, and allow for whole-body breathing. Its impact on our pelvic floor health is immediate. Fortunately, there are a number of techniques that can help you learn to work orally, including certain yoga poses, jaw and tongue stretches, cranial sacral mouth work, and, of course, vocalizing and singing.

### Inquiry and Exercise

- Run your tongue over the palate in your mouth, feeling the palate's dome-like shape. Gently push the tongue around the edges and imagine a widening toward the back of the hard palate and from side to side.

- Then with clean or gloved hands, place your index fingers on each side of the roof of the mouth near the teeth, and with very gentle pressure widen the palate. What do you feel? Does it feel like your whole face is widening? Can you imagine or even sense a parallel widening in the pelvic dome or in the arches of your feet?

- Now keep your tongue wide, but let it "float" in your mouth. What do you feel in the back of your throat, your cheekbones, and the space between your eyebrows? On a very subtle level, the face softens.

- Still keeping the tongue wide, stick it out as far down toward your chin as you can. Reverse the movement and lift it up toward the nose as high as you can. Then move it to the left and to the right. Then, using a paper towel, gently grab both sides of your tongue and softly tug on it. These all help stretch the attachments of the tongue.

  - Press the tip of the tongue against the back of the bottom teeth, and flex the middle of the tongue upwards. For more advanced tongue twisting, you can hold a pen by reaching your tongue over it to increase the arching.

  - Make the sound *mmm* while visualizing the vibration widening the roof of the mouth.

  - Assume lion's pose (*simhasana*), stretching the tongue toward the chin, keeping it long and wide.

### Suggestions from Ann Dyer

- For grounding and creating a dynamic relationship between the tongue and pelvic floor, chant aloud the Sanskrit sound *gam* (pronounced GUM). Now chant *lam* (rhymes with "hum"). The sounds originate at the back of the tongue and activate the pelvic floor in slightly different ways. Can you feel the difference between the two sounds in your pelvic floor?

- Chant the vowel sounds *a, e, i, o, u* one at a time at the normal pitch of your voice for the duration of one relaxed breath. Then gradually drop the pitch of the note and do the same thing. How low can you comfortably go? Can you feel the vibration of the sound lower in the body as the pitch is lowered?

## Core Beliefs

Having looked at the anatomy and the mechanics of the pelvic region, let's explore a place we have all heard of, "the core."

If you practice yoga, Pilates, or Bar Method, you have probably heard the instruction to *work from your core*. Classes are often spiked with catch phrases like "core power" or "core strength." This wouldn't be bad if everyone understood what *core* means. However, if asked to describe the core, most people will wave their hand over their belly area and guess "My front abdominals?"

Like the Loch Ness monster or Bigfoot, the core is legendary and elusive. How can we engage the core properly, if we don't know exactly what muscles are meant to work? This lack of knowledge means we may run the risk of harming ourselves by not working our core correctly. In fact, some of the practices that are billed as "strengthening the core" may do the exact opposite.

We need core muscles for power, strength, and stability. We need to use them when we lift something heavy in order to avoid straining other, more vulnerable parts of the body, like the lower back. We need them to work as shock absorbers, like when we drive too fast over a big bump. We need them to keep our spine and organs safe when we are jumping, dancing, and playing sports. Core muscles are crucial for our stability and safety.

The core musculature consists of

- The diaphragm, which attaches at the xiphoid process (bottom of the breast bone) along the 7th to 12th ribs, and to lumbar vertebrae L1, L2, and L3.

- The pelvic floor muscles, which run from the pubic ramus to the ischial spine, ischial tuberosity (sitting bones), and coccyx with attachments along the crus of the clitoris and perineal body and encircling the anus, urethra, and vagina.

- The abdominal muscles, of which we have four layers. The most superficial layer is the rectus abdominis (the famous "six pack"), which runs vertically from ribcage to pelvis. On the sides of the torso are the external and internal obliques, which run diagonally from lower ribcage to pelvis. The deepest abdominal muscle, the transverse abdominus (TrA), runs horizontally beneath the other layers. Because the TrA is the deepest abdominal muscle and runs in a lateral (side-to-side) rather than a vertical (up-and-down) manner, it is often considered the true core by many in the anatomy world. When the TrA is properly recruited, it works like the cinching in of a corset.

- The postural spinal muscles (multifidus spinae), which extend from C1 (top of the cervical spine) to the sacrum. The short and deep muscles attach between the spinous and transverse processes as well as the vertebral bodies. They are like super-supportive struts.

There are many reasons we fail to engage the full range of core muscles. One of the most common is "perma-tuck" of our bellies—we hold in our bellies because we want to look thin. Perma-tucking has become such a habit that people don't even notice it anymore. Many women have told me their mothers encouraged them from a very young age to keep their belly pulled in to look thinner.

By the way, the social pressure to look thin is a relatively new phenomenon. When we look at sculptures from ancient Greece, or paintings by Rubens or Renoir, we see women with nice soft round bellies. The Gibson Girls were full-figured gals in the early 1900s, and even as late as the 1950s, we still admired the voluptuous body of Marilyn Monroe (I am pretty sure that if Marilyn were a star today, the tabloids would call her fat). Rather than real corsets, we wear mental corsets. I have worked with students who trained themselves to hold their bellies in so strongly that they were unable to take a full abdominal breath. This puts constant strain on the lumbar discs and the pelvic organs.

The perma-tuck is often exacerbated by the instruction to "work your core," which people commonly interpret as "pull your belly in as intensely as you can."

And that brings me to another pet peeve, the "navel to spine" cue. It's true that when we strongly pull our navel toward the spine, a lot of muscles are activated. The problem is that this action also makes our rectus abduminus and erector spinae muscles dominant. The rectus muscle is our most superficial abdominal muscle, but it is not necessarily considered a stabilizer because it also flexes the spine (think forward bends). When we pull the navel to the spine, the pelvis tucks even more and the spine becomes less stable. That action destabilizes our poses and increases the chance for injury, which is the exact opposite of what we want.

If the cue, "draw the navel to the spine" is inadvisable, what are some alternative actions for activating the core?

I prefer phrases like "draw the sides of the navel toward the back of the body" or "draw the frontal hip points toward one another," in order to keep the spine in a neutral position. Overworking the rectus can result in too much spinal flexion, which can make us vulnerable to lower back pain or even nerve impingement. Pelvic health specialist Isa Herrera, M.S.P.T., of Renew Physical Therapy in New York City, asks us to "draw our navel to our heart." Experiment with these cues in your own body and see which one gives you the most stability. Just avoid the "navel to spine" action.

It takes time to learn how to properly stabilize the core. Here is an exercise that *seems* relatively easy. However, you will need to be careful, as the body creates all kinds of ways to cheat.

### Leg Lifts

1.  Lie on the ground. Place a blanket under your head. Bend the knees and place the soles of the feet on the floor.

2.  Place your fingers on the lower belly, below the navel and above the pubic bone.

3.  Lift your feet a few inches off the floor (if you have back pain, lift only one at a time). Observe what happens to the area under your fingers and to your lower back.

Most likely you will feel that your belly muscles firm and lift toward the ceiling. You may also notice that your low back lifts off the floor and begins to overarch. Some people say that their lower back actually flattens. If this is the case for you, put more support under your head.

Now try a variation of this exercise.

Follow instructions 1 and 2. Lift the perineum toward the crown of the head as you exhale (you need to be in neutral to do this). Slowly lift your feet off the ground.

Did you notice a difference in your belly and your back? Most people experience that the belly no longer lifts toward the ceiling and the lower back remains stable; there's no overarching.

The abdominal stabilizers work most efficiently when the pelvic

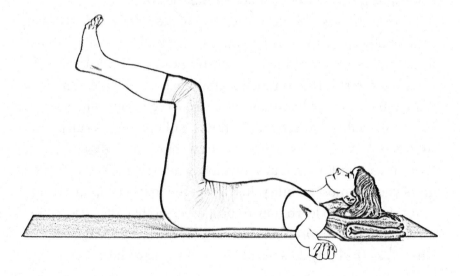

floor is recruited. I have worked with women who were instructed to engage only the transverse abdominus, and they tend to push down on their pelvic floor. However, the instruction to contract the pelvic floor muscles first will help to engage the entire core.

It takes time and patience to learn how to properly work with the various muscles called the core, but doing so is immensely important for a happy, healthy pelvis.

## Neutral Pelvis, Neutral Spine

Having practiced yoga for most of my life, I have heard countless mentions of how to gather my tail and put it under me. Tuck it, scoop it, pull it forward, lengthen it toward the ground—the instructions are infinite.

Then I took a workshop with Judith Lasater. I was happily tucking away in *tadasana*, when she called me out: "Push your femurs back and release your tailbone," she said. "Release your tailbone!" After a few awkward tries, I succeeded. I felt my butt popping out and imagined that it must look like I had a peacock feather tail. "*That* much out?" I thought. It was an eye-opening moment. I could actually breathe better. In retrospect, that was the beginning of my tailbone's liberation.

Pulling your tailbone forward (flexing the coccyx) especially when you don't need to shortens the pelvic floor muscles, putting the pelvic organs at a disadvantage. Loss of the anterior tilt means the organs can't use the pubic arch as a shelf and may become prone to prolapse. When we tuck our tailbones unnecessarily, it overloads the lumbar discs and hampers the spine's ability to work as a shock absorber. We need adequate room between our discs to ensure that the nerves that flow from the spinal column and spinal cord have enough space and don't become entrapped, impinged, or otherwise cause pain.

Ideally, our spine has three natural curves: the lumbar or lower back curve, which is concave; the mid-back or thoracic curve, which is more convex; and the curve of our neck or cervical curve, which is concave again. Any misalignment in one of the curves will force the others to react in kind. And as the spine grows out of the pelvis, the position of your pelvis naturally affects the curves of the spine.

I believe the instruction to tuck your tail is intended to take the pelvis in a posterior direction, which is necessary in backbends and many standing poses. The problem is that literally tucking the tail is not the right approach to getting the whole pelvis to move posteriorly. Inappropriate tucking of the tailbone can carry a number of serious risks. Some people will do a small, localized action at the tip of the tailbone near the anus, but that action will not help keep compression out of your lumbar discs while doing backbends. Instead, take the top of the buttocks away from your lumbar, and draw the front hip points toward the ribcage to keep compression out of the lumbar spine.

Now, some of you are saying: "I am not a tucker. In fact, I have been told by yoga teachers that I have a swayback!" Swayback, or a hyperlordotic back, means too much lumbar curve. Women often tell me that their various instructors (yoga, personal training, ballet) have encouraged them to tuck more to compensate for overarching their lumbar.

Yes, swayback can create serious stress in the area where the pelvis and spine meet (the lumbosacral joint) and on the hip joint. But tucking is not the solution. Strengthening the pelvic floor muscles can often improve a swayback. It is important to develop awareness of where your *neutral pelvis* is (everyone's will be slightly different), which allows the curves of the spine to communicate with each other in an optimal way.

Hyperlordosis is a concern, but it is common for a swayback to be misidentified. There are other, perfectly normal reasons for what may look like hyperlordosis. For example, some women are simply blessed with naturally round buttocks that may give the impression in profile of an extreme curve in the spine. Others have mastered the art of "mothertucking" the pelvis but then they throw their front ribs forward, which also looks like a swayback. I call these people rib-poker-outers or RPOs. When given the instruction to lift the chest, RPOs will often throw their front ribs too far forward, creating shear pressure on the spine.[18]

Now there are students who have swayback because of too much anterior tilt of the pelvis. What's happening in those cases is that the anterior superior iliac spine (ASIS, frontal hip points) is tipped forward of the pubic bone, thus creating a hyperlordosis of the lumbar spine. This can happen because of tight hip flexors, quadriceps, or lower back erectors paired with weak or inhibited abdominal muscles. There are yoga poses that can help.

### *King Dancer Pose (*Natarajasana *Variation)*

Preview: This pose will help to stretch quadriceps, psoas, and the groin area. The mistake I see many students make with this pose is they lean forward and pull the bent leg back too much. The key to deepening the stretch is to keep the pelvis in a more posterior/tucked position.

**How to Practice**

1.  Begin in mountain pose (*tadasana*; page 170) with your feet together and arms at your sides.
2.  Shift your weight onto your left foot, then bend your right knee and bring your right heel toward the outer edge of your right buttock.
3.  Reach your right hand down and hold the top of your right foot. You can also loop a strap around the top of your right foot and hold onto the strap with your right hand.
4.  Draw your inner knees toward each other.
5.  Reach your left arm overhead or, if you need to steady yourself, place your left hand on a wall.

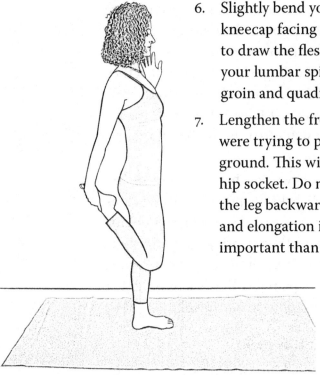

6.   Slightly bend your left knee, keeping the left kneecap facing forward. This action allows you to draw the flesh of the buttocks away from your lumbar spine. Feel the stretch in the right groin and quadriceps.

7.   Lengthen the front of the right leg as if you were trying to put your right kneecap on the ground. This will create space in the right hip socket. Do not yank on the foot and send the leg backward. The traction of the hip and elongation in the thigh muscles is more important than taking the thigh back.

8.   As you press your raised foot into your hand, keep your chest lifted. Do not let your torso drop forward. Keep your pelvis square and your right knee toward the midline of your body.

9.   If you are holding a strap, walk your hand down the strap toward your foot until you can clasp the top of your foot with your right hand.

10.  Hold for 1 to 3 minutes. To come out, release the right foot and return to *tadasana*.

11.  Repeat the pose on the opposite side for the same amount of time.

### Half Reclined Hero's Pose (Ardha Supta Virasana)

Preview: This pose is practiced to open the front of the leg, particularly the groin, quadriceps, and psoas muscles. If this pose is too challenging, stick with the King Dancer Pose until the body opens up a bit more.

**Props**

- Three yoga blocks
- Blanket

**How to Practice**

1. Set up three yoga blocks on your mat. The first one, where your buttocks will be, is on the lowest height. The second is where your shoulder blades will rest and will be on the medium height of the block. The third block is for your head to rest on and can be on either the medium or tall side, depending on your need.

2. Sit down on the first block with your right leg in *virasana* and your left leg bent, foot on the floor, left knee pointing toward the ceiling.

3. Place a folded blanket under the right knee for support.

4. Lie back with your shoulder blades resting on the second block and your head supported on the third block.

5. While in the pose you are working to keep your pelvis in a posterior position to maximize the stretch in the front of the right thigh.

6. Push the left foot into the mat with the intention of drawing the top of the left buttock away from your lumbar spine.

7. Draw the right frontal hip point (ilium) toward the head.

8. Lengthen the right femur bone from the hip socket toward the kneecap. Stay in the pose for 1–3 minutes.

9. To come out, sit all the way up, then switch sides.

**Modifications**

- You can use bolsters and folded blankets instead of the two blocks under the shoulders and head. But sitting on a block helps keep the stretch where you want it.

- If the stretch is still too intense, sit the buttocks on the floor in front of the support of shoulders and head. Practice this way until you can tolerate having a block under the pelvis.

- If the stretch in the front of the ankles is too intense, roll up a blanket to support the area and do the seated version of this pose first.

- If this pose is too challenging, try the seated version of Hero's pose until the muscles open up a little more.

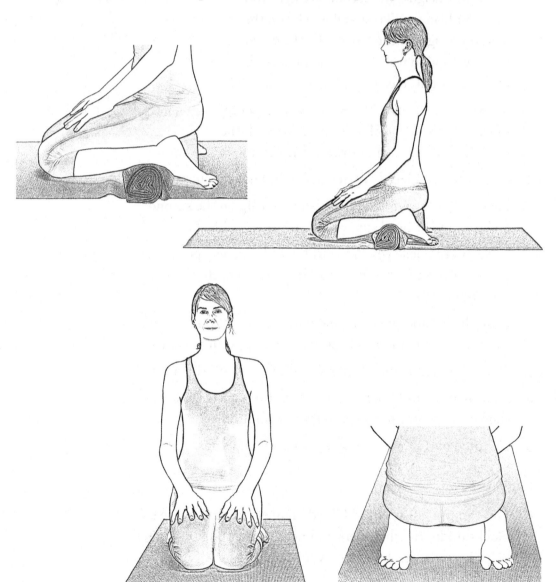

**Focused Actions**

- The two most important actions for the reclined version of this pose are the sense of elongating your right thighbone while keeping the pelvis in a tucking position.

- The tucking of the pelvis is similar to the action of the pelvis in lateral standing poses.

- For the seated version, the primary action is to gently press down through the top of the feet and lengthen both thighs from the hip to the knee (like you are trying to make them longer).

## *Lunge*

Preview: This is a very common pose practiced in most yoga classes. But many students don't take their feet far enough apart to feel a stretch in the back leg. For this pose to be most effective, make sure the stride between the two feet is as long as it can be while keeping the front leg at 90°.

**How to Practice**

1. Start in mountain pose with yoga blocks on either side of your feet.

2. Place your hands on the blocks. Step your right foot back, coming into a lunge position. Make sure your left knee is over your left ankle.

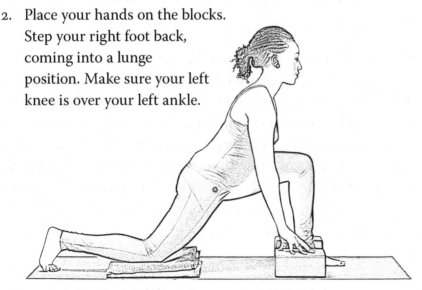

3.  To ensure your stride is correct, move your back foot as far away from the front foot as you can, keeping the right angle of the front knee. This should provide a stretch in the front of the groin or quad in the back leg.

4.  Reach through your back heel continuously as you slowly lower your right knee to the floor. Maintain the stretch in the front of the back leg. Pushing the back heel into a wall can help with this.

5.  With your right knee on the floor and your right toes tucked, push through the right heel as if you were about to lift the knee.

6.  Take your right fingertips to the right glute and notice whether it is engaged or not. If not, contract your right gluteus maximus to keep the right femur head back and stretch the right groin more. Without this engagement, your femur can push forward into the groin area and, over time, cause injury, including labral tears in the ring of cartilage around your hip socket.

7.  Move the right front hip point toward your head and the right buttock away from your head.

8.  Stay in low lunge for 1 to 2 minutes. To release, lift the back knee up and step forward with the right leg.

9.  Repeat on the left side.

As we go about our day, we move through anterior, neutral, and posterior pelvic tilt many times, and that is completely normal. What matters is our ability to return to our "homepage," the neutral pelvis. If we don't know how to do that, we are bound to injure ourselves or to get habitually stuck in a position that will harm us in the long term. Think about it when you are standing in line, sitting in your car, or waiting quietly at the beginning of a yoga class. There are many opportunities for us to "come home" every day.

~

What exactly does it mean to have a "neutral" pelvis? And how can we best find that position?

Most definitions of a neutral pelvis go like this: Your spine is in neutral when the ASIS, known as the frontal hip points in yoga, and your pubic symphysis are on the same level or same plane. In other words, your pelvis is in a neutral position relative to your spine.

This is not a bad description, but it can be hard to apply practically. Some people have very prominent pubic bone and others' are very flat while some have belly fat so the hip points are not easily marked. Others (like me) have been tucking for so long that striving to get the ASIS and the pubic symphysis on the same level would cause pain or aching in the lower back. Some are blessed with a generous butt and will have a hard time finding neutral, especially when supine. Everyone's body is different, everyone's neutral will be a little different.

Let's look at a few ways we can find our neutral. Because there are so many body variables, here are a number of options to help you find the one that's best suited for you.

1. Try this standing. Bring your awareness to the perineum. If your arms are long enough (or your torso short enough), place a finger on your perineum. Imagine that at the spot where the finger touches there is an eyeball. Now overtuck your pelvis (move it posteriorly) so that the imaginary eyeball looks forward. Then really stick your tail out (move it anteriorly), untucking your pelvis so that the eyeball looks behind you. Finally, bring the eyeball of the perineum so that it looks straight down. This is neutral. This exercise also works in a seated position as long as you sit on a firm surface for accurate feedback from your sitting bones.

2. Awareness of the depth of your breath is a good indicator of a neutral pelvis. When standing, keep the legs actively straight, tuck your pelvis (pull your tail under you) and take a deep breath. You will notice that the breath is short and contained in the upper chest. Now reverse the movement—

stick your butt out as much as you can—and take a deep breath. You will feel the breath more in the front of your chest. It may go down a little farther than before, but it still can't move all the way to the pelvis. Finally, play around with finding a position for your pelvis that's between the two extremes, and watch your breath. When you find the neutral middle ground, you will experience the fullest circumferential breath. This exercise also works in a seated position as long as you sit on a firm surface for accurate feedback from your sitting bones.

Note that whole-body breathing happens when we are aligned while sitting or standing in a neutral position. If the pelvis is too far forward or backward, the spine can't reach optimum length. This affects the pump-like movement of our primary breathing muscle, the diaphragm.

Another way to find neutral more easily is if we know how to distinguish the lift of the perineum. If you are new to pelvic liberation, this may be a bit difficult. Review the Meet and Greet section on page 53. Use a blanket if you need padding for your knees.

1. Come onto hands and knees. Place hands directly under the shoulder joints. Place knees directly below the hip joints.

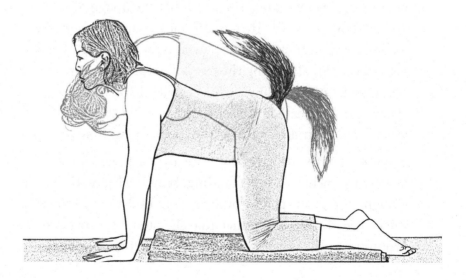

2. Cow: On the inhale, lift the head and the tailbone toward the ceiling, thus arching the back down. Lengthen the front abdominal muscles. Note that when head and tail are up, the pelvic floor is lengthening.

3. Cat: On the exhale, round the spine up toward the ceiling, and draw the sides of the navel toward your spine. Move the head and tail toward one another, rounding the back and tucking the pelvis. When the head and tail are tucked, the pelvic floor is shortening.

4. Following your breath, move between cow and cat for three to five rounds.

5. Find neutral, which will be approximately halfway between cow and cat.

6. Play around with this position by slightly tucking your tail while lifting your perineum; you will feel more of an anal sensation. Then go slightly past your neutral into untuck and lift the perineum again; you will feel the front triangle of muscle in the pelvic floor and/or the vagina and urethra close. Play with this until you develop a sense of the muscles that engage; let the perineum be your guide.

Finding a neutral pelvis while lying down offers a wonderful opportunity to get in touch with the back of the body and to sense some of our spinal habits.

1. Lie down face up on a firm surface with your head supported by a blanket. The knees should be bent, feet flat on the floor. Close your eyes and bring your awareness to the feeling of your back body against the ground.

2. After a minute or two, place one hand on the lower front ribs and the other hand on your pubic bone. Feel into the corresponding areas that are resting against the floor.

3. What do you notice? Are your back ribs firmly on the floor? Are they slightly lifted or strongly lifted? What part of your sacrum is resting on the floor—the top, middle, or bottom?

4.  Tune into where your lumbar spine is in relation to the floor. Is it lightly or firmly against the floor, or perhaps arched away from the floor?

5.  Keeping the back ribs pinned to the ground, bring the mid-sacrum to touch the ground. Your lower back may or may not touch the ground, depending on the anatomy of your lower back and the size of your buttocks. However, this is a good guideline that will help you to find your way to a neutral ribcage, pelvis, and spine. Notice the quality of your breath with this alignment.

~

**Generally change in our society is incremental. Real change, enduring change, happens one step at a time.**

—RUTH BADER GINSBURG,
Associate Justice, U.S. Supreme Court

These wise words from Justice Ginsburg apply to attempts to change the way we inhabit our bodies, too. Whatever our pelvic and spinal habits, they won't change overnight. It is important to remind ourselves that we can't force change upon them. We don't want to risk damaging our lower backs. Finding healthy pelvic and spinal habits is a slow and gradual process. However, finding and experiencing a neutral pelvis can be life-changing—really.

# III | Unhappy Pelvises: Conditions, Cures, and Common Misconceptions

## Conditions

### Incontinence, Prolapses, Varts

Pelvises and families have a lot in common, and one of those elements is nicely summed up in the famous remark that "all happy families are alike; each unhappy family is unhappy in its own way" from Russian writer Leo Tolstoy. Happy pelvises are (relatively) alike, but there are an infinite variety of conditions that can render our pelvis unhappy—or dysfunctional, as they say in family psychology.

Fortunately, many of these conditions fall into general categories, so we can look at a few issues women regularly experience. But we always need to keep one caveat in mind: there can be a lot of individual circumstances associated with each condition; a one-size-fits-all approach rarely works.

The most common pelvic issue for women is incontinence, and that can take a tremendous toll on quality of life. It can cause shame, fear, and even depression. Women who experience incontinence may go into the world with serious fears: Where's the nearest bathroom? What if I can't make it to a bathroom in time? Can other people tell if I've leaked? Even if the condition isn't debilitating, it can seriously curb activities that once brought joy. I have talked with runners, weightlifters, and self-described gym rats who felt they had to give up their passions because of fear of urinary leakage. Moms and grandmothers may be afraid to play too vigorously with the kids or might avoid going on long road trips. Urinary incontinence impacts *life.*

According to the Centers for Disease Control, more than one-half of non-institutionalized women in the U.S. age 65 and up reported urinary leakage in a national survey of more than 2,600 people.[1] In addition, a 2011 analysis of nearly 64,000 U.S. women aged 36–55 determined that 13.7% of women who reported no or minimal leaking developed at least monthly incontinence over the next two years, corresponding to an average incidence of 6.9% per year. At the same time, only 38% of those in the study with frequent incontinence mentioned their urine loss to a physician, and only 13% reported receiving treatment.[2]

As the study cited above shows, many women don't tell their doctor about this issue.[3] They may believe that urinary incontinence is a long-term side effect of having given birth, a symptom of menopause, or simply part of aging. If they do tell their doctors, sometimes they get a shrug and a "prescription" for—surprise, surprise—Kegel exercises.

~

There are many forms of incontinence, but the most common are caused either by stress or by urge. Stress here refers to something that works as a stressor on your pelvic muscles, such as coughing, sneezing, laughing, running, or jumping. The leakage associated with stress incontinence often happens without any forewarning, as there is sometimes no sensation of having to urinate. Stress incontinence is generally (but not always) associated with a lack of muscle tone in the pelvic floor (hypotonic muscles).

In contrast, urge incontinence is associated with clear sensation. In its early stages, urge incontinence produces a strong feeling of needing to urinate immediately without leakage. Just walking by a bathroom may be enough to conjure up that urge to go. Giving in to urge incontinence potentially sets up a faulty brain-bladder connection where the desire to urinate occurs even if there is little or no urine present. An easy way to check if your bladder is truly full is to keep a log of your need to go and how long your urine stream is. If you feel the urgent need to go, but your urine stream goes on for less than ten seconds, the bladder is not full.

As the condition worsens (sometimes aggravated by Kegeling), "key in the door" syndrome may occur, whereby a person is able to hold their urine with uncomfortable and overwhelming urge for a while (maybe the ride home) but when getting to their front door or bathroom door experience leakage.

Urge incontinence is often due to overly tight (hypertonic) pelvic floor muscles. If urge incontinence is left unaddressed in its early stages, it may progress to the point where urine escapes before the person makes it to the bathroom. It seems counterintuitive but the solution is to relax your pelvic floor muscles.

If you are suffering from stress or urge incontinence, it's good practice to keep track of your liquid intake, your bathroom patterns, and what can trigger urination (like coffee, tea, or acidic drinks). It's even more important to not lump the different forms of incontinence together; stress and urge incontinence have different causes and different manifestations. Usually, they require different therapeutic approaches. When someone with hypertonic pelvic floor muscles has symptoms of urge incontinence, she needs to learn to relax the pelvic floor, which can lessen the urge sensation, or even make it go away. For someone with stress incontinence, learning how to stabilize and firm the pelvic floor muscles can vastly improve symptoms. It's important to differentiate the two types of incontinence or we run the risk of engaging in a course of treatment that may make matters worse.

So is it possible to have both stress and urge incontinence? Unfortunately, the answer is yes, and this is called mixed incontinence. Here is a common example: A new mom carried a babe in her womb, supported by her pelvic floor, for nine months. She then went through a prolonged labor. Post-birth, she wants to get back in shape and goes to the gym. But after the "butts and guts" class, she finds that she has gotten herself "wet and upset," and experienced stress incontinence. She resolves to remedy this and, having read about Kegel exercises, starts doing as many as she can each day. To avoid any further accidents, she does a "preemptive pee" anytime she leaves the house. Her brain-bladder connection goes awry and tells her that any amount of liquid in the bladder signals "find a bathroom." Urge incontinence begins. Between the Kegeling and the urgent trips to the bathroom, she is now someone whose pelvic floor muscles are too loose and too tight, but in different areas. If this sounds familiar, it is crucial to address the urge symptoms first.

Another common condition is pelvic organ prolapse. This is when a pelvic organ "falls" from its usual position into the opening of the vagina. Remember, in the female pelvis, the bladder sits toward the front, the rectum toward the back, and the uterus is nestled between the two. While all three organs can prolapse, it occurs most commonly with the bladder, according to various sources, although hard data are tough to come by.[4] In some cases, the prolapse is so severe that the bladder or uterus may hang outside of the vagina. Some women manage this situation by simply pushing the prolapsed organ back in, or by wearing something called a pessary to hold things up. A pessary is similar to a diaphragm and can be inserted and removed by the wearer. If the bladder prolapses, it's called *cystocele*; if the rectum slips forward into the opening of the vagina, it's called *rectocele* and can cause defecation problems. Fortunately, strengthening the different muscles groups of the pelvic floor and maintaining a neutral spinal position can significantly lower the risk of prolapse.

If an organ falls from its usual position, it's easy to blame a lack of strength. But pelvic organ prolapse (POP) can also occur if the ligaments holding the organ in place have overstretched or sustained damaged. POP can also be a result of a chronically tight pelvic floor after a prolonged battle with chronic constipation. Straining to defecate can contribute to or cause POP, as well as hemorrhoids. Don't make assumptions about the status of your pelvic floor without further investigation or help from an experienced pelvic floor specialist.

Here's a question I often get asked—usually whispered to me at the end of the workshop—"What about varts or queefs?" A "vart" occurs when air is taken into the vagina and suddenly released with the sound of passing gas (though without odor). This happens usually as a result of going upside down and may cause embarrassment when it happens in a crowded yoga class. It is usually an indication of low tone in the vaginal walls.

Hypotonicity, or low tone in the pelvic muscles, can have any number of different causes. One of the most common is excessive bodyweight exerting constant pressure on the pelvic muscles. While the obesity epidemic is a topic of public discussion, most of it centers on the impact of excess weight on cardiovascular health, or on the bones and joints. But excess weight has tremendous impact on our pelvis, stretching out the muscles to the point where they have low or no tone. Note that weight gain during pregnancy can also stretch out and strain the pelvic muscles.

## More Conditions

Let's look at some of the more common issues associated with hypertonic or overly tight pelvic muscles. There are many things that may indicate tight pelvic muscles, such as urinary frequency or urgency; a change in urination, such as slow or delayed stream; or a feeling of not emptying the bladder fully. Problems with defecation are another sign, such as pain leading up to, during, or after a bowel movement, or even a change in bowel frequency. But the first indicator is often pain in the pelvic area.

### Vulvodynia

A Latin word that means "pain of the vulva," which is the external female genitalia, vulvodynia can sometimes feels like a yeast infection with typical symptoms of burning or itching; irritation caused by tight clothing; or discomfort during many forms of exercise, such as biking.

According to the National Vulvodynia Association, there are many causes and factors contributing to this complex condition:

- An injury to or irritation of the nerves that transmit pain from the vulva to the spinal cord

- An increase in the number and sensitivity of pain-sensing nerve fibers in the vulva
- Elevated levels of inflammatory substances in the vulva
- An abnormal response of different types of vulvar cells to environmental factors, such as infection or trauma
- Genetic susceptibility to chronic vestibular inflammation, chronic widespread pain, and/or inability to combat infection
- Pelvic floor muscle weakness, spasm, or instability

### Vaginismus

A painful spasmodic contraction of the vagina, vaginismus some-times occurs in response to physical contact—say, when inserting a tampon—or the fear of physical contact, perhaps in the context of attempted sexual intercourse. In severe cases, the opening of the vagina starts to close involuntarily. The resulting pain can be mild to searing. While there is some uncertainty about the causes of vaginismus, the condition does result in the superficial layers of the pelvic floor contracting to become short and tight.

Many women blame themselves, but vaginismus is rarely a controlled or voluntary condition. There may be physical or non-physical reasons for it. Frequently women very much want to achieve penetration and they don't understand why they can't. This condition can be very stressful for women and their partners. Relaxing and stretching the pelvic floor muscles may help relieve the symptoms of vaginismus.

### Lichen Sclerosis (LS)

An autoimmune disease of uncertain origin, the primary symp-tom of LS is itching (although not always) and small white patches on the skin of the vulva, clitoris, vestibule, anus, or belly. While hypertonic muscles in the pelvic floor do not directly cause LS, there is an association between the condition and tight pelvic floor muscles.

Due to the pain, itching, and discomfort of LS, the pelvic floor muscles contract to guard the area, which can exacerbate the pain and discomfort. Learning to relax the pelvic floor can sometimes help to alleviate LS symptoms.

### *Irritable Bowel Syndrome (IBS)*

IBS may be associated with hypertonicity of the pelvic floor. IBS commonly causes cramping, abdominal pain, and bloating. The disorder is often marked by periods of constipation and then colon spasms that result in diarrhea. Some women tend more toward constipation and some more toward diarrhea. The exact cause of IBS is unknown, but the disorder may be related to tightness or dyssynergia (muscles contract when they should be lengthening), causing difficulty in defecation. If you experience new onset of bowel symptoms, you should see a healthcare practitioner before seeing a pelvic floor P.T. for a pelvic floor muscle assessment.

### *Interstitial Cystitis*

Also know as painful bladder syndrome, interstitial cystitis often feels similar to a urinary tract infection. It can cause an overwhelming urge to urinate, frequency of urination, or pain and burning with urination. But going to the bathroom results in only a weak stream and the urge to urinate remains. Note that this is different from urge incontinence where there is a short stream but the bladder does empty. Inability to empty the bladder completely can lead to urine retention and painful ulceration of the bladder lining and can cause great pain. If the pelvic floor muscles are tight and unable to relax fully, they won't allow the bladder to empty completely. One way to manage these symptoms is to consciously relax the pelvic floor muscles while voiding. If that proves difficult, then do a "double void." First, empty the bladder as much as possible, then change your position on the toilet (i.e., lean your torso forward and tilt the pelvis more anteriorly) relax the pelvic floor, and see if the stream starts again. This is preferable to leaving the bathroom and then coming back a few minutes later.

Taking a look at your bathroom habits can help. It is important to sit down and relax when urinating so that the bladder empties completely. This is why it's best not to do the "hover," or what I call "public bathroom *utkatasana*." When you hover over the toilet seat, the muscles of the pelvic floor contract and send a seriously confusing message to the body. "Hold me up and also relax and pee at the same time?" It is much better to sit down on the toilet. Now, I know many of us protest, "Have you seen the public bathrooms at Grand Central station?" Yes, I have. But studies have shown that we are more likely to catch a virus or bacteria from the light switch or door handle in a public restroom than from contact with toilet seat.[5] You can always use the disposable paper toilet ring, or wipe down the seat with an antiseptic wipe before you sit down. But take a seat and allow your pelvic floor to relax.

Remember, having one or any of these conditions doesn't automatically mean that you are fully hypertonic or hypotonic. The pelvic floor is complex, so both conditions may be present. In addition, tone can fall anywhere on a spectrum, so we may be really tight on one side and a little too loose on the other. The main message is that we need to carefully assess our conditions and choose the appropriate therapeutic measures to address them.

## Cures

Hopefully by now you see that there is no one-size-fits-all approach to address pelvic floor health. It follows that we need to question exercises and devices that are promoted as universal panacea for all pelvic issues. Just Google remedies for various pelvic health issues and you'll notice the lack of differentiation.

### Kegels

Let's look at some of the standard "cures" that are often suggested for pelvic floor issues, such as Kegel exercises. The practice of "Kegeling" gives truth to the saying that if all you have is a hammer, everything looks like a nail. If the only tool you have to address pelvic health problems is squeezing everything tight, then loose is all you perceive. Now there is a role for Kegel exercises for pelvic health. But it's just one tool, which cannot, and should not, be used across the board. It may even be harmful when used inappropriately. You wouldn't use the hammer to fix the delicate heirloom tea set you inherited from your grandma, would you? We need to recognize our conditions and understand which tools are best for us. Let's look at some pelvic grievances.

> **Kegel** [key-guhl] verb—squeezing everything from the navel to the knees and hoping for the best, as defined by Leslie Howard.

When I ask my students to define Kegel exercises, they most commonly describe it as performing a contraction that stops the urine flow. There is a vague but general consensus that it involves squeezing down there. But what exactly is being squeezed and for what purpose? That's where things start getting murky.

The exercise was developed by Dr. Arnold M. Kegel, a Los Angeles–area obstetrician and gynecologist. He wanted to develop a remedy for a problem he had noticed in many of his patients: laxity of the vaginal walls and incontinence after childbirth. He had his patients practice *vaginal* contractions, pre- and post-childbirth. In 1948, he devised the "Kegel perineometer," a pelvic-muscle sensor to measure the efficacy of these voluntary muscle contractions. The perineometer was essentially a biofeedback machine. It used a vaginal sensor and an air-pressure balloon that measured the air pressure inside the vagina and verified that the Kegel exercise was being performed correctly.

Over the decades, Dr. Kegel's exercise for strengthening the vaginal walls has become the "go-to" remedy for any problem of the female pelvis. Indiscriminately squeeze "down there" for any and all pelvic floor issues, whether it's appropriate or not.

Let's go back to the description of Kegels being the action of stopping urine flow. This definition is problematic on several levels. If we are told to find the muscles that cut off urine flow, we are more than likely to think of one section of the pelvic floor; what actually stops urine flow is the urethral sphincter, located toward the front of the pelvic floor. This sets up a neural pathway in our brain that exercising the pelvic floor muscles is something that takes place more in the front, which may or may not be where your problem is. So if you've dutifully done your Kegels thinking they are about stopping your urine stream, but haven't seen any results, it may be because you are exercising the incorrect area for you. Don't worry, you are not alone.

This lack of knowledge about how to perform Kegels correctly often extends to the healthcare professionals who prescribe the exercises. A patient may be told that the best way to practice a Kegel is to stop the urine stream at midpoint. Please don't do that! That can lead to urine retention. Proper Kegeling takes time, effort, and a nuanced understanding—it's not something that can be easily understood from the brochure that the nurse hands you on the way out of the exam room. Just finding the pelvic floor muscles, unlike much larger muscle groups like hamstrings or gluteus, requires subtle awareness and training.

So what is correct Kegeling? It engages the pubococcygeous (PC) muscle. The PC is part of the levator ani, and the levator ani muscle group is part of the pelvic diaphragm. In turn, the pelvic diaphragm is part of the larger set of pelvic muscles. Get the picture? Doing a proper Kegel engages only one component of a large team of muscles. Just like in team sports, it won't help if you focus on one all-star muscle, because for optimal performance you need the whole team working in a coordinated way.

There is nothing wrong with practicing vaginal wall contractions if and when it's suitable. I thank Dr. Kegel for his insights and early dedication to women's pelvic floor health.[6] In his day, he was a pioneer in the field.

### *Root Lock (*Mula Bandha*)*

In the yoga world, there is a parallel to Kegels, and this concept is often conveyed in an equally murky way. It's called *mula bandha*.

The history of *mula bandha* is a checkered one. Sri K. Patthabi Jois, an Indian yogi credited with introducing *ashtanga vinyasa* yoga to the Western world, claimed that he possessed an ancient, sacred document called the *Yoga Korunta*. This document allegedly contained the entire series of asanas (postures) and bandhas (locks) of *ashtanga vinyasa* yoga, including a full description of the mechanics and purpose of *mula bandha*. When pressed to produce the text, Jois, claimed the only existing copy had been eaten by ants. He passed away in 2009.

Fortunately, other yoga texts mention *mula bandha* and have not fallen prey to voracious insects. Chapter 3, verse 61 of the *Hatha Yoga Pradikipa*, a 15th century yoga text, instructs the student to "press the heel against the perineum and contract it firmly." But there are no details about the specific muscles that are to be engaged in this description. It's the same with other texts that mention *mula bandha*. In short, there is no *Mula Bandha for Dummies*.

*Mula bandha* roughly translates from Sanskrit as "root lock." The anatomical location where it is performed, the "root," is often considered a seat of power, a grounding site for the subtle energies of the body. The ancient Chinese Chi Gung refers to the root lock as "closing the gates" to retain youth and vigor. The essential idea is that we can achieve supreme health and vitality by keeping energy concentrated at the center of the physical body. In the *Hatha Yoga Pradipika*, *mula bandha* is described as a way to "awaken this goddess who is sleeping at the entrance of the *bhahma dwar* (the great door)."

## Misconceptions

If you've been to a yoga class, particularly one in the *ashtanga vinyasa* style, you have probably heard the instruction to lift or engage *mula bandha*. That instruction might be followed by a mention of the perineum or the descriptive instruction to "lift the space between the genitals and the anus." But sometimes the instructions are imprecise and don't explain how to perform this action effectively. As a result, some students may translate *mula bandha* to simply mean "squeeze your ass."

This is unfortunate and hardly conducive to "awakening the goddess" in us. Even worse, it can render *mula bandha* a source of physical and emotional harm. It's like clenching your jaw; if you habitually grind your teeth at night, your dentist wouldn't tell you to engage your jaw muscles more. Instead, she'd likely suggest wearing an apparatus to relax the jaw and to soften that general area. If you already hold tension in the pelvic region, then creating more tension through Kegeling or *mula bandha* is inappropriate, and can possibly cause pain. It comes as no surprise to me that I encounter a lot of yoginis with hypertonic pelvic floor muscles.

One general misconception that drives Kegeling and *mula bandha* is that becoming loose "down there" is inevitable, either post-birthing or because of time and age. Subsequently, we are told that we need to do something to combat this laxity. But as we learned earlier, a pelvis that holds too much tension can be as much of a problem as one that is too loose. Recognizing these misconceptions, and the potential harm they can cause, requires an understanding of body mechanics and energetics. From there, we can develop a yoga asana practice that accommodates and adapts to our diverse bodies.

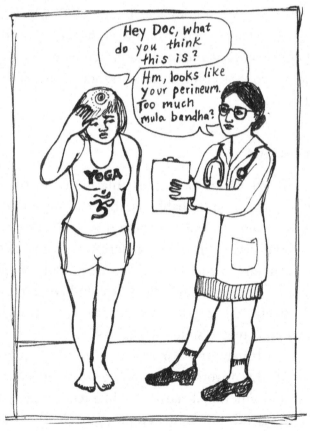

# IV | Yoga: Help Is on the Way

## Why Yoga?

Many people with pelvic issues attend my workshops after having tried a number of different approaches to deal with them, often consulting first with their general practitioner, then a gynecologist, then a urologist. They may have tried Kegels, muscle-building exercises, or even antidepressants. Some have reached a point where they are considering surgery.

Let's look at this scenario: A woman in her mid-40s starts feeling pain during intercourse. Her doctor recommends using more lubricant, but that doesn't help. She visits a gynecologist who can't diagnose a reason for her painful intercourse. She starts to read about the issue on the Internet, which offers exercises that may solve the problem. She does the exercises but they don't help. She starts to wonder if her symptoms are psychosomatic and seeks a psychotherapist . . . The list goes on.[1]

Each of the approaches above (allopathic medicine, exercise, counseling) has its merits. But for many women, yoga is the last resort. I've worked with women as a yoga teacher for over 20 years and as a pelvic floor yoga teacher for over 12, so I say this with absolute certainty: Yoga should be the first resort. Here's why.

Practicing yoga cultivates self-awareness and sensitivity toward your body; it isn't just another set of exercises you do. Yoga fosters subtle observation and awareness of your body's mechanics and energetics. It gives you experiential insight into the unique form and shape of your individual embodiment. It allows you to understand what is happening as it is happening, and gives you the tools to adjust your practice to constantly fluctuating conditions, moment by moment. It is one thing to have a general conceptual understanding of the anatomy of muscles; it's something else to be able to locate, sense, and work with the individual muscles in your own body.

Body awareness is key to properly diagnosing ailments. No doctor in the world will be able to tell you what it's like for you to feel pain or tension or relief or any other sensation; this is information only you can access. This type of insight is critical to making a proper diagnosis. Yoga combines external conceptual knowledge with the internal experiential understanding that only you can access.

Yoga is empowering. It empowers you to take an active role in your own healing rather than handing over responsibility to a doctor or someone else. It encourages and supports you to see for yourself. After all, it is your body, and you should not blindly give up control. You hold primary authority over your body, and you need to exercise that authority by exploring, observing, and learning about yourself. Yoga helps you shed your self-imposed states and empowers you to emerge, to mature, and to take responsibility for yourself.

Yoga provides tools for the healing of many conditions. Both the hypertonic and hypotonic pelvic floor can often be effectively remedied with yoga. Yoga provides a complex and nuanced set of tools you can fine-tune to address your specific circumstances in a non-invasive, holistic way. In addition, yoga is compatible with and complementary to internal physical therapy.

The world of yoga stretches wide and deep in many directions. You can use it to explore and address a particular issue, or you can embrace it more fully and let it carry you to a transformative life.

In this chapter, we will look at yoga poses with the intent of addressing specific pelvic conditions. As you practice these poses, I encourage you to pay attention to the specific energy each of them carries. Poses are often experienced as calming, invigorating, focusing, heating, cooling, and so on. When you understand the energy of different poses and how they affect you, you can use this knowledge to energize, balance, and calm your life; to challenge yourself; to cultivate greater sensitivity and compassion; or to simply enjoy a richer and much more complex range of sensations and emotions.

## Getting Started

My intention is to create an accessible way to focus on the technical, precise, and sometimes subtle instructions that can alleviate pelvic floor challenges, so that even the beginner can understand how to approach the poses for maximum benefit. Some of the poses build strength and help us find and contract the muscles. Some lengthen the muscles, while others soften the muscles. Some focus on the breath.

I have separated the poses into two categories to address hypertonicity and hypotonicity. The poses are presented from easiest to more challenging, but not in a specific sequence for a particular symptom. Hopefully you have done some of the diagnostics suggested in the book and you know whether you need to do the poses for hypertonic or hypotonic pelvic floor. Remember if you are a combination of both you need to address the tight muscles first. Getting chronically tight muscles to let go can sometimes happen rather quickly or in some cases may take up to a year (that is how long it took mine to let go).

If you found the muscles were too tight, you need to practice:

- daily whole body breathing
- posture vigilance (standing and sitting)
- daily (or nightly) internal massage
- poses to relax and stretch the pelvic floor

Once you feel like your pelvic muscles have let go, I encourage you to alternate with the poses in the hypotonic section because those are geared toward stability and strength. We all need mobility and stability.

If you know you are hypotonic and your pelvic floor muscles are weak or non-responsive, you need to practice:

- daily whole body breathing

- posture

- positions to differentiate your perineum, your urethral and anal sphincters, and your vaginal walls

- pelvic floor contractions (both quick and longer holds) several times a day and in different positions (standing, sitting, supine, prone, all fours)

- poses to strengthen and stabilize

I have created sample sequences for particular issues, which begin on page 231. However, everyone's pelvis is so different. I strongly encourage you to experiment with the poses and see how you and your pelvis respond.

If your life schedule permits, establish a routine that will make it easier for you to practice yoga at home. For example, it can help to practice at roughly the same time and in the same place each day. Practicing with someone else may make it easier or more fun to do your yoga exercises at home. But remember that poses are designed to help you address a particular health challenge and get you more in touch with your body. Practicing alone and in a quiet space can open you up to continual inquiry: What am I feeling? How is my breath? Where do I feel movement created by the breath in each particular pose?

Don't push yourself in the early sessions. Remember that some yoga postures are more difficult to maintain than others. Be patient with yourself. If you are feeling tired after practicing some of the more challenging postures, switch to practicing supported legs up the wall pose (page 202) or supported lying down bound angle pose (page 160) for 10 minutes. With practice, you should find it easier and more relaxing to assume and maintain all of these postures. If there are specific poses that you find more challenging to practice, vary them with postures that you find easier or more relaxing.

Doing yoga postures should not lead to breathlessness—this indicates that you might be a reverse breather (see box on page 52), or that the pose is too challenging for now. Either try the pose with more support or try the pose at another time. The heart of practicing yoga postures is to train the nervous system to be calmer, even in a physically challenging pose. The breath will always let you know if you are doing too much.

### Yoga Props

To help you practice yoga at home, invest in a yoga mat, one yoga strap (at least 8 feet in length), two foam blocks, a couple of sandbags (8–10 pounds each), two or three yoga blankets (yoga blankets are firm cotton or wool), a bolster, and a timer. If you can, keep your yoga props in plain view so they remind you to take time to do your practice.

You don't need to spend money on props if you've got a tight budget. Items around your house can also serve as props:

- Firm bath towels or bed blankets can be used in place of yoga blankets

- Large, firmly rolled towels or firm sofa cushions can be used in place of yoga bolsters

- Books can be used in place of yoga blocks

- Belts or neckties can be used in place of yoga straps for many of the poses. Note that there are a few poses for which a yoga belt that can fasten into a loop will be beneficial.

- If you use the timer on your phone, put it in airplane mode while practicing so you are not tempted to check your email while in *baddha konasana* or *shavasana*. I suggest using a traditional cooking timer instead.

- For those with knee challenges, putting a rolled up washcloth behind the knee can help, so you may want to have one handy.

## YOGA AND BREATHING
### for Hypertonicity

### *Relaxation Pose with Weight (Shavasana)*

Preview: This setup is the same as for *shavasana* (relaxation pose) which is done at the end of your practice, but weights are added to promote a focus on inviting the breath to go deeper and more fully into the lower torso. Remember, deep breathing helps the pelvic floor stretch on the inhale and contract on the exhale. The stretch should not happen because you are manipulating the muscles; the positive effect on the pelvic floor happens as a result of better breathing. From our inquiry on whole-body breathing on page 55, we know that most students can detect that they breathe differently in their two lungs and that each lung expands at a different rate on the inhale. We will begin from the place where we were breathing more into the belly and pelvic floor.

### Props

- Three blankets: one folded for under the head, one rolled for under the knees (or a bolster under the knees works too), one folded to put across your thighs

- Strap if you have issues with sacral instability

- Two yoga sandbags, 8–10 pounds each. *Note:* If you use a weight plate (20–30 pounds) instead, use an extra yoga mat to secure the plate on top of your legs

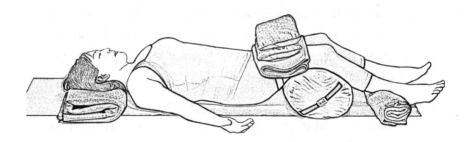

- Optional:
    - Blanket to cover yourself
    - Rolled blanket for under the Achilles tendon
    - Yoga eye pillow or scarf to place over the eyes

**How to Practice**

1. Place your mat on a firm surface (don't do this on the bed) with the folded blanket that will serve as a pillow for your head ready on the mat.

2. Sit on your mat with a bolster or blanket under your knees.

3. If you are using sandbags, place them directly on your mid-thighs. *Note:* If the sandbags feel cold, place a folded mat or blanket across your thighs and put the sandbags on top of that. If you tend to get cold, cover your body with an extra blanket.

4. Lie on your back with the legs extended and arms at your sides. Rest the arms about 6 inches away from the body with the palms up.

5. Let the legs relax. Close the eyes.

6. Invite the breath to travel into the belly and lower back. Note that the movement of the breath in the chest may become less pronounced as a result.

7. Imagine the body releasing toward the ground.

8. Consciously release every body part, organ, and cell, starting from the soles of the feet and moving to the crown of the head.

9. Relax the face. Allow the eyes to drop deep into the sockets. Stay in the pose for 5 to 20 minutes.

10. To exit the pose, bring your awareness back to your body. Use gentle movements and wiggle your fingers and toes. If you are using the sandbags, pull them off the thighs.

11. Roll on to your right side. Rest on your side for a moment.

12. Press the left hand into the floor, letting it do the work to help bring you into a comfortable seated position.

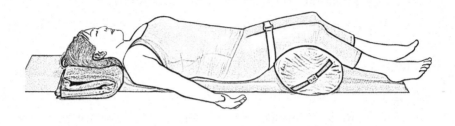

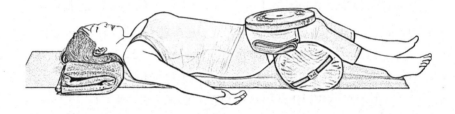

**Prana *and* Apana Vayu**

According to Yogapedia, *prana* is a Sanskrit word that has a number of interpretations in English, including life force, energy, and vital principle. *Vayu* is a Sanskrit word meaning wind. *Prana* is subdivided into five *vayus*.

The *prana vayu* is one of the five energy subdivisions of *prana*, and is considered one of the most important. It is situated in the head and is considered the fundamental energy. *Prana vayu* is responsible for the reception of everything into the body from air to food, senses to thoughts. Being aware of the *prana vayu* is vital for obtaining optimal benefit from yogic practices, as the movement of *prana* throughout the body is the essence of yoga.

*Apana* is the second-most important of the five *vayus*, particularly for Hatha yoga and Ayurveda medicine. *Apana vayu* is responsible for regulating the outward flow of *prana* from the body. It governs the elimination of physical wastes and toxins from the body. Located in the pelvic floor, it spreads upward into the lower abdomen, helping to regulate digestion and reproductive functions.

SOURCE: yogapedia.com/definition/8518/apana-vayu, accessed July 6, 2017.

**Shavasana** *Variation with* **Apana Vayu Mudra**

Preview: The word *mudra* translates from the Sanskrit as a seal (as in an energy seal, not the animal). Mudras are commonly done with the hands. *Apana* energy in the body flows downward. But it can get blocked for many reasons. We need clear *apana* energy for good digestion, elimination, and menstruation, and for more easeful births. Too much tension in your pelvis will keep the *apana* energy from flowing as well as it could. This mudra can help deepen the breath and calm anxiety.

1. Follow instructions for *shavasana* and whole-body breathing. Add the *apana vayu mudra.*

2. Start with an open hand. Fold the index finger into the mound of the thumb. Gently place the thumb on top of the index finger to keep it in place.

3. Join the tips of the thumb, middle finger, and ring finger.

4. Extend the pinky.

5. Extend the arms with the hands 6–8 inches away from the torso.

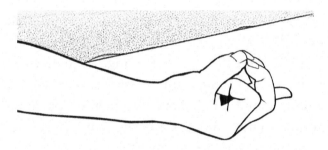

*Bumblebee Breathing* (**Bhramari***)*

Preview: Bumblebee breathing helps quiet the mind. The intention is to fill the body with sound and vibration to quiet our constantly chattering inner voice. Bumblebee breathing can be done on its own or paired with *shanmukhi mudra. Shanmukhi mudra* is when you lightly place fingertips and fingerprints on eyes, ears, nose, edges of the lips to quiet the senses.

**Props**

- Folded blanket, bolster, or block to support the sitting bones in neutral while sitting on the floor. You can also do this pose while seated in a chair or lying down.

**How to Practice**

1. Sit in any comfortable position so that you are on your sitting bones. Your pelvis should be in a neutral position.

2. Rest the hands with palms up in the lap or on the thighs.

3. Gently press the sitting bones down into the support. Lift the crown of the head toward the ceiling. *Note:* To help with this action, imagine balancing a book on the crown of the head and push up into it to elongate the spine upward.

4. Slowly, bring the chin back and in, so that the underside of the chin is parallel to the floor.

5. Close the eyes and take a few slow, deep breaths. Consciously relax all the muscles of the face and forehead.

6. Inhale deeply through the nose.

7. On the exhalation, make a humming sound like that of a bumblebee buzzing around. The exhalation will occur naturally as a result of the humming. The humming vibration should come from the back of the throat. The humming sound should have a deep or low pitch. If the humming sounds high pitched, the sound vibration is coming from the top of the mouth.

8. You want to sound like a bumblebee, not a mosquito. Keep the sound soft and consistent. Feel the vibration in the top of the head, the palate, and maybe even the pelvic floor.

9. Exhale completely, inhale again deeply through the nose and repeat the bumblebee breath.

10. Breathe like this for 1–5 minutes.

## *Bumblebee Breathing with Six-Gate Mudra* (Brahmari *with* Shanmukhi Mudra)

Preview: *Shanmukhi mudra* quiets the senses to increase the calming effect of *brahmari* pranayama. The six gates refer to the openings of the ears, nose, and eyes. This mudra creates a withdrawal from the senses (state of *pratyahara*) that promotes a meditative state of mind. Please note, you might not want to do the mudra if you have long fingernails.

### How to Practice

1. Raise your hands to your face so that your arms are at shoulder level. Place the tips of your thumbs in the earholes so that surrounding sounds are muffled. Then, lightly place the fingerprints/pads of the index fingers on your upper eyelids, the tips of the middle fingers on the inner corners of your eyes, the tips of the ring fingers on the outer notches of the nostrils to narrow the nasal passages, and the pinkie tips on the outer corners of the mouth.

2. The touch of the fingers on the face should be very soft. The intention of your hands is to widen the face energetically, which means you are not actually pulling on the face but visualizing doing so.

3. Begin *brahmari* breathing, keeping the pitch of the hum low.

4. Focus on the vibration created by the exhaling hum extending out from the back of the palate toward the ears so that it has a wide quality rather than a vertical quality. Practice this for 1–3 minutes.

### Modifications

- If the arms get tired doing *shanmukhi mudra*, use an eye wrap instead of the hand mudra.

### *Bumblebee Breath with Eye Wrap (*Brahmari *Variation)*

Preview: The eye wrap is made of soft cotton with a very small amount of elasticity in it. You can order these online through most Iyengar Yoga Centers. Some teachers say you can use an ace bandage, but I think that creates too much pressure in the head. The wrapping of the head creates a withdrawal from the senses (state of *pratyahara*) that promotes a meditative state of mind.

**How to Practice**

1.  To use the wrap, start with the roll intact and lightly hold the loose end of it to one temple. Unwind the wrap as it goes over the ears and around the base of the skull.

2.  When you've unwound the whole roll, tuck in the end.

3.  Find your seat or your setup for lying down.

4.  Once you are settled with all the props you need, you can pull the eye cover over the eyes and begin your bumblebee breathing.

5.  Breathe like this for 1–5 minutes.

6.  To come out of the pose, either slowly unwrap the head or gently take the wrap off using your fingers near the base of the skull to draw it up and off the head.

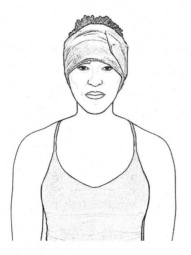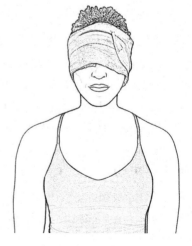

## Poses for Hypertonicity

### *Staff Pose (*Dandasana *Variation)*

Preview: A strap provides support while seated with the pelvis in a neutral position (on the sitting bones) and helps you get familiar with the feeling of working the legs properly. The strap keeps the legs very active and prevents you from falling back into a slumped position with a rounded low back. While this pose can be done without a strap, it is most effective with one.

#### Props

- Strap, fastened into a large loop
- One to two blankets

#### How to Practice

1. Sit on the floor with the legs straight in front of you, in line with the hips. The torso should be 90° to the legs. If your hamstrings are tight, sit on a blanket to keep the pelvis in neutral.

2. Take the looped strap over your head and place the loop mid-buttock and then around one heel. The loop should now be held in place with the mid-buttock and the heel.

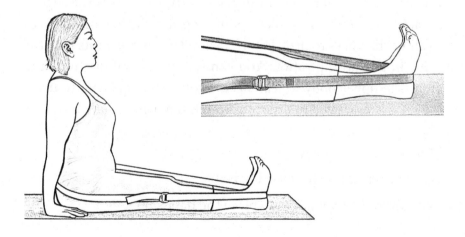

3. Adjust the strap until it is snug enough that you have something firm to push into, but not so tight that you cannot fully straighten the leg.

4. Press into the loop with the heel by elongating the whole leg. Do not let the heel lift off the floor as this will cause the knee joint to hyperextend.

5. Push the inner leg and inner foot into the loop. Gently pull the little-toe side of the foot toward the outer hip. Notice the effect of the pose with the looped strap. You may find the looped leg feels closer to the ground. There may be more space at the top of that hip socket. You may find that the breath flows more freely on the looped side.

6. Remain in the pose for 1–2 minutes.

7. To come out of the pose, release the strap.

8. Repeat with the other leg.

### Modifications

• If you need to sit on a lot of height to maintain a neutral pelvic position, you may want to use a thinly rolled blanket under the backs of the knees to prevent hyperextension.

### *Bound Angle Pose (*Baddha Konasana*)*

Preview: Use support under the pelvis, sitting on either the edge of a stack of several firm blankets or on a bolster. Sitting high enough to allow the knees to drop below the level of the hip joints puts the spine in a neutral position. You can set up in front of a wall and allow the upper body to lean against the wall. For hypertonicity, the pose is practiced in order to stretch the pelvic floor.

### Props

• Bolster or two to three blankets

• Optional: two blocks to place the hands on

**How to Practice**

1.  Sit on a bolster or folded blankets, possibly against the wall. Your imaginary tail should be behind you. Reach the crown of the head toward the ceiling. The perineum should be parallel to the floor.

2.  Bring the soles of the feet together (if this is difficult, see Modifications below). Let the right knee drop to the right and the left knee drop to the left.

3.  Keep the feet together. Bring them as close to the pubic bone as you can.

4.  Ensure that you are still sitting equally and evenly on the center of your sitting bones.

5.  Place the hands on the edges of the bolster or blankets (or blocks if you have them, see illustration below) behind the pelvis. Push into the hands to lift through the crown of the head.

6.  Stay in this pose and keep pushing with the hands for 3–5 minutes.

7.  To come out, place the hands on the outer knees and gently draw the knees in toward each other. Straighten the legs and return to *dandasana*.

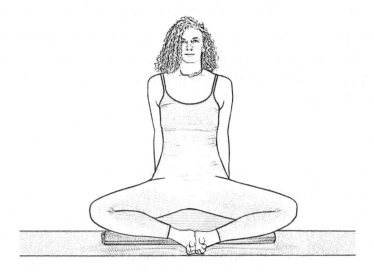

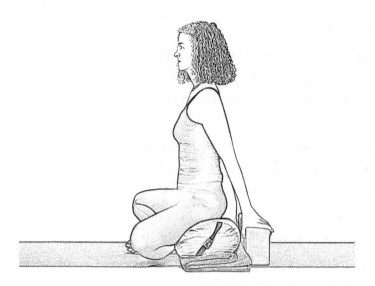

## Modifications

- If the hips and groin are tight and it is challenging to bring the soles of the feet all the way together, start with the outer edges of the feet together.

- To prevent the heels from coming apart, keep the ankles slightly flexed, particularly the outer edge (i.e., little-toe side) of the foot.

- If you experience knee pain while practicing this pose, place a rolled up washcloth behind the knee (between the back of the thigh and calf) to create more space behind the joint.

- To avoid pelvic floor muscle contraction, lengthen through the inner groin (topmost part of the inner thigh) toward the inner knee. Alternatively, remain passive in the legs. Focus on the breath.

## Focused Actions

- There can be a tendency to fall back in the pelvis so that the lumbar spine rounds and the pelvic floor contracts (i.e., tucking the pelvis). Manually adjust the flesh of the buttocks behind the sitting bones; that is, grab each buttock and pull the flesh out from under the sitting bones.

- Keep the little-toe edges of the feet together. Lengthen from the perineum to the inner knee, as if someone were gently pulling the inner thighbone away from the hip socket.

### *Reclining Big Toe Pose 1 (*Supta Padagushthasana 1*)*

Preview: This supine posture stretches the hamstrings. Tight hamstrings can contribute to tight pelvic floor muscles. If practiced with attention to the placement of the lumbar spine and a neutral pelvis, it can help lengthen the first and third layers of the pelvic floor. A second yoga strap can be used to create traction at the hip socket and awareness of the relationship between the bottom leg and the opposite hip, as described in the Going Deeper section at the end of this pose instruction.

### Props

- Blanket

- One to two straps (second strap is optional and needs to be 10 feet long)

### How to Practice

1. Lie supine on the floor with your knees bent, feet on the floor, head on the folded blanket.

2. Check that your lumbar spine has its natural curve. (For most people, there will be a little bit of space between the low back and the floor.)

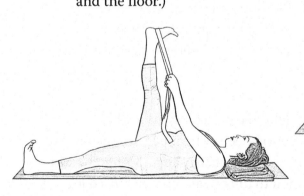

3. Draw the bent right knee toward the torso. Interlace the fingers around the shin or back of the thigh. Gently hug the thigh to the belly.

4. Place the strap around the right sole, just where the front heel meets the arch.

5. Straighten the right leg, reaching the right heel toward the ceiling. Emphasize the push of the foot up and into the strap. The strap is there to give the leg something to push into. *Note:* Don't pull the leg toward the head as this flattens the lumbar curve.

6. Lengthen the back of the left (bottom) leg along the floor. Push through the left heel. Don't push so strongly that the heel lifts off the floor as this is a sign of knee hyperextension. *Note:* Imagine releasing the tail toward the floor. This will help the pelvic floor muscles elongate. The weight of the body against the floor is not on the lower back but more toward the sacrum and tail.

7. Work the legs by reaching into the heels and pressing the heels away from the hips. Notice the breath. You may find that breathing into your belly and pelvis is easier on the left side.

8. Keep the right leg vertical (in the air) for 1–3 minutes.

9. To come out, bend the right knee to the chest. Remove the strap. Bring the leg in the line with the hip. Lower the right leg next to the left. Relax both legs for a few breaths.

10. Before doing the left side, notice the breath. Are there any differences between the left and right sides? Then notice how the legs feel. Does one leg feel lighter, longer, warmer?

### Modifications

- If the hamstrings are tight, the pelvis may tuck when straightening the raised leg. Keep a slight bend in the knee of the raised leg. For hypertonicity, it is more important to keep the pelvis in neutral than to fully straighten the raised leg.

- If holding the leg vertical for 2–3 minutes causes excessive fatigue, hold the pose for less time. Instead, do the pose multiple times on each side, resting in between.

- If your low back hurts, bend the knee of the bottom leg.

- It is counterproductive to take the leg past a 90° angle, even if that is in your capacity. This sharp angle will cause the pelvis to tuck and will tighten the pelvic floor muscles, further aggravating your condition.

### Focused Actions

- Ensure that the lumbar spine is not pushed into the floor. The weight should rest more on the mid-sacrum. Make sure the back ribs have not lifted off the floor. Ideally, the lumbar spine is lightly resting on or slightly away from the floor and the back ribs are touching the floor. This will help maintain a neutral pelvis.

### Going Deeper

- Take the second yoga strap and make a large secured loop. Place it around the heel of the bottom leg and the hip crease of the top leg (See illustration below).

- On the bottom leg, press more through the inner leg and inner heel. This will pull the outer hip of the lifted leg and create more length in the spine.

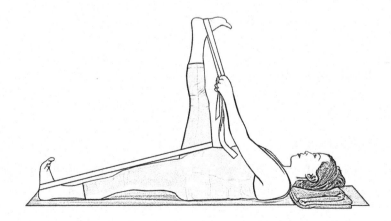

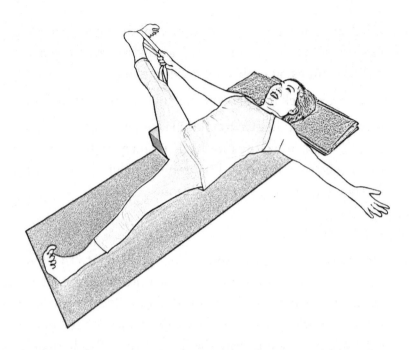

### *Reclining Big Toe Pose 2 (*Supta Padagushthasana 2*)*

Preview: The previous pose focused on stretching the back of the leg. This pose focuses on stretching the adductors (inner thighs) to lengthen the second layer of the pelvic floor. The origin of some of the hip adductors (particularly the gracilis) is where the anatomical legs of the clitoris insert. Stretching the adductors can sometimes alleviate difficulty in attaining orgasm (that should get you doing this pose).

### Props

- Blanket for under the head
- Strap
- Block or bolster

### How to Practice

1. Start in *supta padagushthasana* 1.

2. Place a soft yoga block, a bolster, or a firmly rolled blanket up against the outer edge of the right hip socket.

3.  Place the strap around the right foot where the front heel meets the arch.

4.  Take both ends of the strap into the right hand and straighten the right elbow, holding the strap as close to the foot as possible with the shoulder still on the floor. The bottom leg is straight.

5.  Rotate the right leg out so that the toes point away from the torso. *Note:* Remember that the foot turns as a result of the external rotation of the hip, so make sure you are turning the head of the thighbone, not just the foot.

6.  Take the right leg out to the right and toward the ground. Support the outer thigh on the block or bolster.

7.  Once the leg is out to the side, extend from the groin toward the inner heel.

8.  Remain in this position for 1–2 minutes.

9.  To come out, bring the leg back up toward the ceiling. Bend your right knee to the chest. Lower the right leg next to the left. Relax both legs.

10. Before repeating on the left side, notice the breath and any differences between the sides. Notice the legs; does one leg feel lighter, longer, and warmer? Does the hip socket feel more spacious?

## Modifications

*   If you find yourself tipping to one side, press more strongly into the heel of the bottom foot. If this isn't enough, set yourself up facing a wall and press into the wall with the foot of the leg that is on the floor.

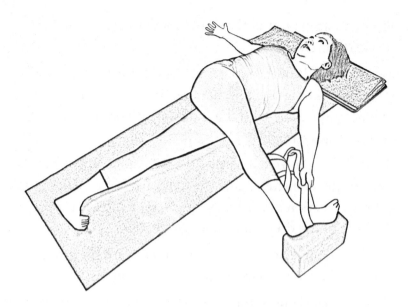

### *Reclining Big Toe Pose 3 (*Supta Padagushthasana *3)*

Preview: The previous pose focused on the inner leg. This pose focuses on the outer hip and leg and stretches the abductors and IT (iliotibial) band. It will also stretch the hip rotators like the piriformis and the gluteus medius. I wish I could say it helps with orgasm too but that would be yoga propaganda.

#### Props

- Blanket for under the head
- Strap
- Block or bolster

#### How to Practice

1. Place a support (block or bolster) about one leg length away from your left hip at hip level.

2. Starting from *supta padagushthasana* 1, take the right leg up with the strap around the foot. Hold the strap with the left hand, near the right foot.

3. Cross the right leg over to the left, placing the right foot on the support. This will stabilize the hip joint.

4. Keep both legs straight and active. Turn the chest and head to the right.

5. The lumbar spine should not round.

6. Stay in the pose 1–2 minutes.

7. To come out, turn the chest back to the center. Bend the right knee, release the strap, and roll to lie flat on your back. Compare your two sides before moving on. How do your hips feel? How is your breath on each side?

8. Repeat on the left side.

**Modifications**

• Support the entire raised leg, not just the foot, on a bolster.

• If your hamstrings are tight, bend the right leg slightly to prevent rounding in the lumbar spine.

**Focused Actions**

• Draw the outer foot (little-toe side) toward the outer hip (remember the action in staff pose).

• Gently push thighbone of the bottom leg into the floor and lift the thighbone of the top leg toward the ceiling. This action helps widen the top of the sacrum.

### *Half Happy Baby Pose (*Ardha Ananda Balasana*)*

Preview: This pose facilitates a stretch in all the pelvic floor muscles. The difference in the tightness of the hips is usually more obvious in this pose than in the ones you have done so far, and this will inform you of possible imbalances.

**Props**

• Blanket

• Optional: one block (use if you have discomfort in the hip crease when doing this pose)

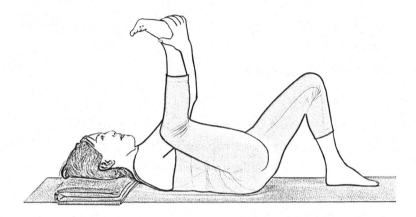

**How to Practice**

1.  Lie on your back with the head well supported. Take a little more support than you would usually as this will make it easier to release the tailbone. Bend the knees, with the soles of the feet on the floor.

2.  Bring your right knee toward the chest. Reach between the legs and take hold of the little-toe side of the right foot with the right hand.

3.  Bring the sole of the foot parallel to the ceiling, ankle over the knee so the shin is perpendicular to the floor. Flex through the heel.

4.  Keep the knee lined up with the armpit (think upside down lunge). Lengthen the right sitting bone away from the head. This is the same as unfurling the tail.

5.  Keep the ankle over the knee so that your shin stays perpendicular to the floor.

6.  Bring your attention to the sacrum and tailbone. Release the tip of your tail toward the ground as if you were unfurling it. *Note:* The weight on the sacrum will be slightly heavier on the right but try to minimize this. If you bring your thigh too far out from the side of the torso, the weight will be all on the right side of the sacrum.

7.  Remain in this pose for at least 1 minute; try to work up to 3 minutes.

8.  To come out of the pose, release the foot to the floor and rest.

9.  Repeat on the left side.

**Modifications**

•   If it is too challenging to hold the foot, grab the ankle or calf. Or use a strap as an arm extender and loop the strap around the foot. Hold the strap as close to the foot as you can. You also can take the knee slightly wider than your body, but don't let the knee swing out too much from the body.

•   If the tailbone is very tucked into the body and you can't release it closer to the floor, take additional support under the head.

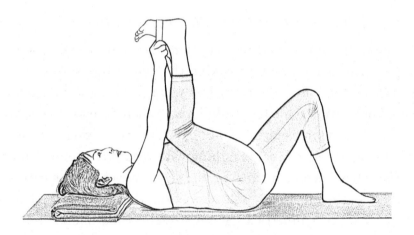

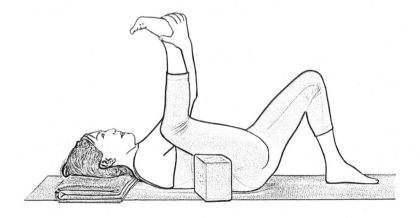

- If you feel compression or discomfort in the groin, place a block between the thighbone and the floor to keep space at the top of the hip socket.

**Focused Actions**

- Don't push the low back strongly into the floor and curl the tailbone toward the ceiling. Instead, imagine unfurling the tail. This will alleviate weight on the lumbar spine. Draw the tail away from the head. The more you can take weight toward the bottom of the sacrum, the more the first and third layers of the pelvic floor can stretch.
- As you are holding the right foot, hug the right knee in toward the body and draw the right sitting bone away from the left. This will stretch the second layer of the pelvic floor.

### Dynamic Tabletop (Cat-Cow, Tail Wag, Hula Hoop)

Preview: This pose has three variations. First, in cat-cow, you will experience tucking and untucking the pelvis; this shortens and lengthens the pelvic floor muscles from pubic bone to tailbone and from sitting bone to sitting bone. When doing cat-cow, you will be linking movement and breath. This is an exaggeration of what happens in normal breathing with regard to the movement of the pelvis. Second, in tail wag, the pelvis moves from side to side and is lengthening the muscle fibers from the center to the left or to the right (asymmetrical lateral stretch). Hula hoop combines the two.

**Props**

- Blanket for padding the knees
- Optional: two blocks

**How to Practice**

1.  Tabletop: Come onto the hands and knees with the pelvis in neutral, hands directly under the shoulder joints and knees directly below the hip joints, tops of feet flat on the floor.

2.  Cow: On the inhale, lift the head and the tailbone toward the ceiling and arch the lower back. Lengthen the front abdominal muscles. Note that when head and tail are up, the pelvic floor is lengthening.

3.  Cat: On the exhale, round the upper spine toward the ceiling and draw the sides of the navel toward your spine. Move the head and tail toward one another. Round the back

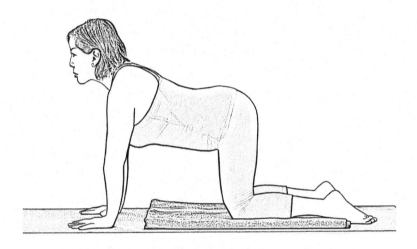

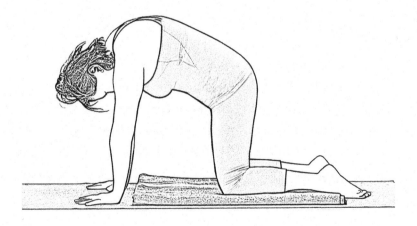

and tuck the pelvis. When the head and tail are tucked, the pelvic floor is shortening.

4.  Move between cow and cat three to five rounds. Move with the breath.

5.  Return to tabletop.

6.  Tail Wag: Move the pelvis side to side to wag the tailbone. When the pelvis moves side to side, layer two will be stretched.

7.  Do the tail wag for 1 minute (see if your family pet comes to give you a few tips).

8.  Return to tabletop.

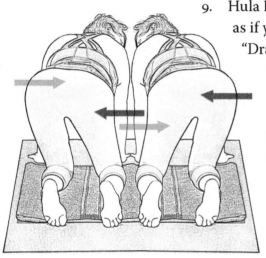

9.  Hula Hoop: Move your hips in slow motion as if you had a hula hoop around your hips. "Draw" circles with the navel on the floor below, or draw circles with your tail on the wall and floor. Make this movement slow and deliberate, not fast and jerky. Note that this movement combines the pelvic tucking and untucking of cat-cow with the side-to-side movements of tail wag.

10. Move in one direction for 1 minute and then reverse the direction for 1 minute.

**Modifications**

*   Rest your forearms on blocks if you have any problems with the wrists being at a 90° angle. Alternatively, use a foam yoga wedge or thinly folded blanket or mat to elevate the heels of the hands higher than the fingers and reduce angle of flexion in the wrist or make gentle fists and lean on your knuckles.

*   If you have severe pelvic pain, don't curl your tail strongly in cat.

**Focused actions**

- Imagine what your pelvic muscles are doing as you circulate your hips (visualize stretching and contracting).

## *Child's Pose (*Balasana*)*

Preview: This pose is a forward fold and a resting pose. It's also a good butt stretch. Generally, this pose is practiced with toes together, knees slightly apart. However, this variation prevents the back from rounding. Remember when the tail is strongly tucked under and the lumbar spine rounded, the pelvic floor muscles are shortening. In this variation, the sides of the torso rest on the thighs or a bolster and the big toes are slightly apart.

**Props**

- Bolster to support the torso and head
- Two blankets, one to cushion the knees and one between heels and buttocks
- Two blocks for the hands

**How to Practice**

1. Start on hands and knees with the bolster beneath you longways, in line with the spine.

2. Bring the big toes about 2 inches away from each other, tops of the feet on the floor, and the knees a bit wider than hip distance apart. Place a folded blanket on the heels. Sit the buttock back on the heels.

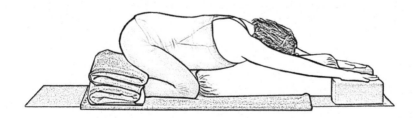

3.  Adjust the bolster so that it supports the ribcage but will not restrict the movement of the breath in the abdomen.

4.  Extend the arms forward and place the palms on the blocks. Gently press the hands into the blocks.

5.  You can turn your head either way, whichever is more comfortable, but if you have neck issues, use a folded blanket or towel to support the forehead so that the head can be straight.

6.  Remain in child's pose for 1–5 minutes.

7.  To exit the pose, walk the hands in till they're in front of the knees and push with the arms to come up.

## Modifications

•   If the buttocks do not reach the heels, place an extra folded blanket (or blankets) between the top of the heels and the buttocks, and/or between the torso and the floor.

## Focused Actions

•   With every inhalation, invite the breath to come into the sacrum and the back of the pelvic floor. With every exhalation, visualize tension leaving the body.

•   To help softly stretch the pelvic floor muscles, the sitting bones should be pointing away from the head, not down toward the floor. Putting enough support on top of the heels can help this.

## *Lunge with Circular Movement 1* (**Anjaneyasana** *Variation 1*)

Preview: This is a modified lunge that creates more space in and around the hip joint. Lunges gently open the hip joint and groin area, both of which can be tight in many people with pelvic pain.

### Props

- Two yoga blocks
- Blanket, for under the knees

### How to Practice

1. Come onto the hands and knees. Place the hands on the blocks.

2. Step the right foot forward to the outside of the right hand. The right foot is slightly turned out and the shin and thigh are at 90°.

3. Press the inner right heel firmly into the floor.

4. Similar to the movement in Hula Hoop, imagine that you have a pencil in your navel and draw circles on the floor, moving the pelvis in a circular motion. It should feel like you're moving the pelvis around the femur (thighbone) head. Remember to keep the head and tail in neutral.

5. After 1 minute, change the direction of the circle.

6. Rest in child's pose before coming to the second side. Notice if the two sides of the pelvic floor feel different.

7. Repeat on the left side.

### Modifications

- If you have wrist pain, elevate the forearms on blocks so that the wrist joint is not at a 90° angle.

- If you feel discomfort in the knee pressed against the floor, put a blanket under the knee.

- If you have any history of sacral instability, make the circular movements smaller. Don't turn the front foot out as much.

- Keep the back knee in line with the hip.

### Focused Actions

- Draw the front leg sitting bone away from the knee to keep the pelvis in neutral.

## *Downward Facing Dog (*Adho Mukha Svanasana*)*

Preview: The flexion of the hips (forward bend) in this pose typically pulls on the ischial tuberosities (the sitting bones) if the hamstrings are tight (and really, who doesn't have tight hamstrings?). This makes it difficult, if not impossible, to get the sitting bones and tailbone to lift. Our goal is to stretch the pelvic floor muscles in this pose, so you will need to bend the knees. This enables you to slacken the hamstrings and therefore untuck the pelvis. We will begin with straight legs so that you can (hopefully) feel difference in your ability to move the pelvis when bending the knees.

### Props

- Optional: yoga blocks or a chair if you cannot tolerate weight on the hands

### How to Practice

1. Come onto the hands and knees.

2. Place the hands a whole hand length (about 6 inches) forward of the shoulder joint. The hips should be directly over the knees with the pelvis in an untucked position, as in cow.

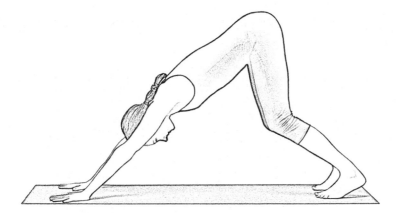

3. Tuck the toes and lift the knees off the floor.

4. Strongly pull the hips away from the hands. Extend through the tail and sitting bones, lifting them toward the ceiling.

5. Push the thighbones back by engaging the quadriceps (front of the thigh) and draw the pelvis away from the torso, straightening the legs to start.

6. Keep the ribcage stable (don't be a rib-poker-outer!). Don't let any extra weight fall into the hands.

7. Now bend the knees. *Note:* The bend in the knees slackens the hamstrings and brings concavity to the lumbar spine. The tailbone and sitting bones can then move away from the shoulders and toward the ceiling.

8. Spread the fingers and ground down into the hands, especially into the thumb mound and root of the index finger.

9. Keep the ears in line with the inner arms.

10. Rotate the thighs inward and push the hips up toward the ceiling and away from the arms.

11. Stay in the pose for 20 seconds to 2 minutes.

12. To come out, bend the knees and rest in child's pose.

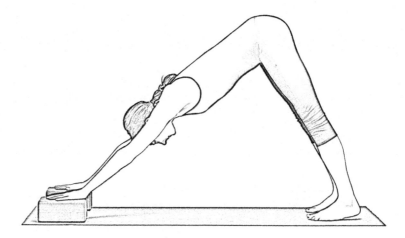

**Modifications**

- If this pose is challenging to hold, you can elevate the hands on yoga blocks. This will help take some weight out of the shoulders. Placing your hands on a chair placed against a wall, or on the wall itself, takes even more weight out of the wrists and shoulders.

**Focused Actions**

- To achieve maximum stretching of the pelvic floor, always keep a bend in your knees to lift the tailbone and increase the lumbar curve near the sacrum.

- Be careful that you are not pushing your lower front ribcage toward the floor. The lower ribcage is where there is the

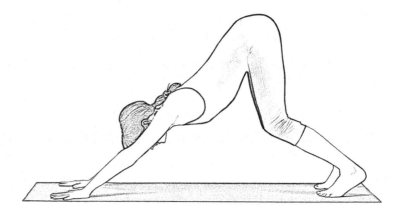

least resistance in the vertebrae. Many people overstretch in the front ribcage without achieving any movement in the lumbar spine and pelvis.

### Mountain Pose (Tadasana)

Preview: This is an extremely important pose because it can improve your general standing position in life. It is a template for all of the standing poses. There are many ways to practice mountain pose. A good way to connect feet, legs, and pelvic floor is to do the pose while holding a yoga block between the upper thighs. This variation teaches the neutral position of the spine (normal curvature; no flat back) and pelvis, so that pelvic floor muscle function is maximized. This pose takes work—don't be fooled into thinking you're just standing around!

**Props**

- Yoga block

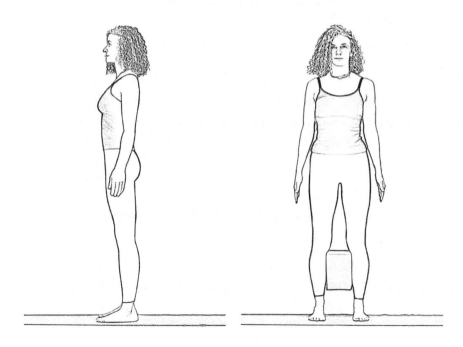

**How to Practice**

1. Stand up straight with your feet slightly apart.

2. Place the yoga block on its narrowest width so that the faces of the block touch the upper inner thighs.

3. Stand with your weight distributed evenly between the feet from side to side, but with a bit more weight in the heels than in the balls of the feet.

4. Find neutral so that the center of the perineum is parallel to the floor and in line with the crown of the head. *Note:* You might feel like you are sticking your tail out more than you are used to. This could be a good sign if you tend to be a mothertucker.

5. Rotate the thighs inward slightly so that the block rolls back. This action creates space on the sides of the tailbone and spreads the sitting bones.

6. Release the top rim of the buttocks down, away from the lower back. Note this is a release and not a tucking action.

7. Lift the quadriceps muscles to lift the kneecaps. This action moves the thighbones deeper toward the back of the leg (hamstrings).

8. Notice how the breath changes with these actions.

9. Lift the crown of the head away from the perineum.

10. Place the arms at your side, palms facing the thighs, fingers together. Steadily lengthen the whole arm toward the ground.

11. Remain in this pose for 1–5 minutes.

**Modifications**

- Practicing the pose with your back against a wall will help you feel the proper alignment.

- If you have flat feet, place the block between your calves (instead of your thighs) and gently hug the block, so that your arches lift.

## Focused Actions

- Push into your inner heels and the mound of the big toe to get lift through the inner thigh. Then lift the center of the perineum to the crown of the head.

- Be mindful not to let your tailbone tuck under you or to allow the thighbones to come forward and roll out.

### Goddess Pose

Preview: Goddess pose is a variation of fierce pose, which is more commonly known as chair pose (*utkatasana*). It strengthens the lower body, stretches the inner thighs, activates the gluteus muscles, encourages the breath into the abdomen, and stretches the pelvic floor muscles when the pelvis is held in neutral. This pose can be done dynamically—with the breath—or statically.

### How to Practice

1. Start in mountain pose. Step the feet 2–3 feet apart.
2. Turn the feet out slightly.
3. Stand with hands on hips, pelvis in neutral.
4. Place weight in the inner heels.

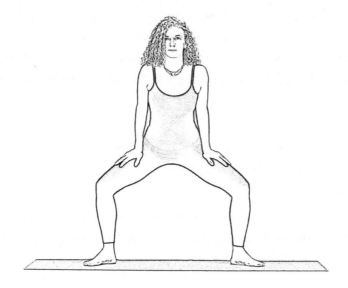

5.  Keeping the perineum parallel to the floor and the spine in neutral and as upright as possible, slowly bend the knees until the thighs are almost parallel with the floor so that the kneecaps face away from each other.

6.  Hold steady for 10–30 seconds, or move dynamically with the breath for 30 seconds to 1 minute (inhale on the way down, exhale on the way up).

7.  To come out, strongly push into the heels, straighten the legs, and bring the feet together.

### Modifications

*   Hold onto something solid (like the kitchen sink).

### Focused Actions

*   Be mindful not to let your tailbone tuck under you, or to allow the thighbones or knees to roll in. When you are bending your knees, the pelvic floor is stretching; when you come back up, the pelvic floor is contracting.

### *Wide-Legged Standing Forward Bend Pose* (Prasarita Padottanasana)

Preview: The aim of this pose is to stretch the pelvic floor by taking the pelvis into an untucked position (anterior tilt). It also stretches the hamstrings without straining the back. If the hamstrings are very tight, this pose is more accessible than Downward Facing Dog.

### Props

*   Two yoga blocks or a chair, as needed

### How to Practice

1.  Start in mountain pose in the middle of your mat facing one of the long sides. Set two blocks in front of you about shoulder width apart.

2. Separate the feet 3–4 feet; set them parallel to each other.

3. Push down on the inner and outer heels and the balls of the big toes. Lift the inner arches of the feet.

4. Folding at the hips, bring the hands to the floor with straight arms and a neutral spine. Keep the length from pubic bone to navel (don't round the back). Keep the head in line with the spine, ribcage in neutral.

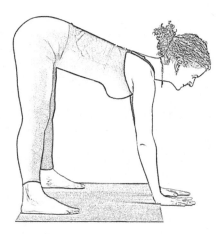

5. Lift the hamstrings to the sitting bones while spreading the sitting bones away from each other.

6. Lift the tailbone toward the ceiling.

7. To come out of the pose, bring your feet under your hips and with straight legs, hinge up to standing.

**Modifications**

- If your hamstrings are very tight, or if getting your hands to the floor isn't possible, use either the blocks or a chair under the hands. Alternatively, bend the knees slightly.

**Focused Actions**

- Visualize the pelvic floor muscles stretching with each inhalation (the breath is being received into the pelvic floor).

- Roll the upper inner thighs internally to soften the groin and widen the sitting bones. This action comes from the hip joint. Be careful not to roll the knees in.

- Make sure your arms are straight and positioned under your arm sockets. Adjust the block height or chair to accommodate this.

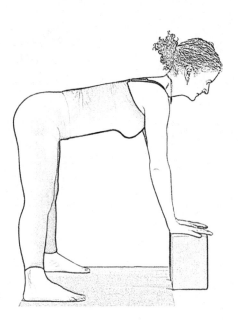
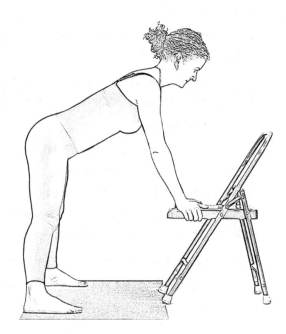

### *Lunge on a Chair* (**Anjaneyasana** *Variation 2)*

Preview: This pose helps create space in the hip joint via a small tractioning action. This will help gently stretch the pelvic floor muscles. Lunges open the hip joint and groin area, both of which can be tight in many people with pelvic pain. This pose is most effective with a strap but can also be done without a strap.

**Props**

- Chair
- Strap, fastened in a large loop

**How to Practice**

1. Stand in mountain pose about 6 inches away from the front edge of the chair seat.

2. Step onto the loop with the left foot, placing the foot so the strap is under the arch-heel juncture.

3. With your left foot on the loop on the floor, bring the right leg through the loop and place the right foot onto the chair seat so that the right leg is at a right angle. The knee should be in line with the heel.

4. Adjust the loop so that it runs under your left foot around your right leg, deep into the right hip crease (not on top of the thigh). Ensure the strap is taut, but not so tight that you can't lean forward.

5. Place the hands on the chair backrest and fold forward from the hips with a long front spine. Don't round the upper back to go further forward.

6. If you have the flexibility to keep the spine in neutral, bring the hands to the chair seat.

7. Keep the left leg active by pressing the inner and outer heel into the floor and lifting the kneecap.

8. Press the ball (more than the heel) of the right foot into the chair seat to keep the right knee in line with the right hip socket.

9. Draw the right sitting bone away from the knee and lift the tailbone, even if you don't feel anything happen.

10. Stay in this pose for 1–3 minutes.

11. To come out of the pose, keep the left leg active. Bring your torso upright.

12. Step the right foot out of the loop and off the chair to return to mountain pose.

13. Before doing the left side, stand on both feet and feel how much more space there is in the right hip socket. Walk around for 30 seconds and notice the difference in the two sides.

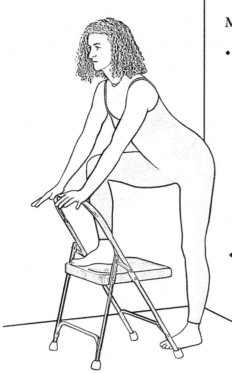

### Modifications

- If you feel unsteady, place the chair sideways in a corner to lean on and set yourself up so that your standing leg is nearer to the back wall.

### Focused Actions

- The lift of the tailbone toward the ceiling helps untuck the pelvis, which stretches the pelvic floor.

- When using a yoga strap, the quadriceps of the raised leg will initially firm. You will feel this as a gripping in the groin. Think about relaxing the quadriceps. If you can do this, the strap will sink deeper into the groin. The pose will become more effective for creating space around the head of the femur.

### Standing Pigeon with Support
### (Eka Pada Rajakapotasana *Variation*)

Preview: This pose is more commonly practiced on the floor. But the standing variation can be more effective for the hip, as well as more accessible for folks with knee issues. It also helps keep the spine closer to neutral rather than rounding the lower back. This pose opens and lengthens the pelvic floor muscles and is a deep stretch for the hip rotators (outer hips).

### Props

- Chair or table (kitchen table height works well)
- Bolster
- One to three blankets

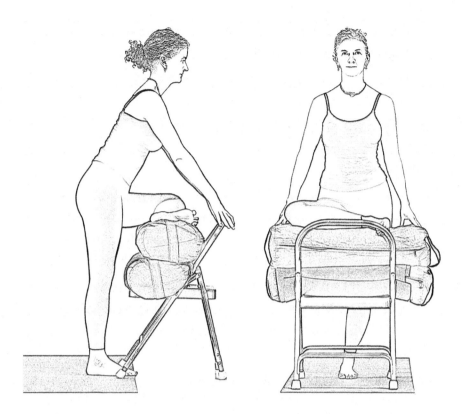

**How to Practice**

1. If using a chair, set it up so that the bolster sits across the seat of the chair the long way. Use two bolsters or enough folded blankets so that the stack is approximately the height of the hip joint.

2. Stand in mountain pose in front of your chosen leg support (the chair with bolster, a table).

3. Keep the left leg in mountain pose.

4. Bend the right knee in front of the chest and turn the right femur out.

5. Place the entire lower leg on the table or the bolster and blankets on the chair seat.

6. Keep the right shinbone parallel to the floor. If the knee is higher than the foot, place extra support under the knee. The shin and thigh of the raised leg should be as close to 90° as your hip socket will allow.

7.  If you can go farther, hinge at the hips and bend forward. Keep the spine in neutral without the back rounding.

8.  Place the hands on the chair back or table surface and elongate the front of the spine as you come forward.

9.  Stay in the pose 1–2 minutes, then change sides.

### Modifications

*   If you experience any knee pain in the bent leg while practicing this pose, use your hand to externally rotate the thighbone more or put support under the outer knee. Alternatively, place a rolled up washcloth behind your knee.

*   The height of the support is determined by the height of your pelvis when standing. You can build up the table height with blankets if you are taller or stand on a yoga block if you are shorter.

*   If you are using the chair variation, you may want to wrap the bolster in a yoga mat to reduce the possibility of it slipping.

### Focused Actions

*   Strongly flex the bent-leg ankle (this helps protect the knee also), so that the outer ankle doesn't overstretch.

### *Supported Bridge Pose (*Setu Bandhasana Sarvanghasana*)*

Preview: This restorative version of the bridge pose is done with support to encourage relaxation and movement of the respiratory diaphragm.

### Props

*   Yoga block

### How to Practice

1.  Lie on your back with the block nearby.

2.  Bend the knees to 90° with the soles of the feet on the floor.

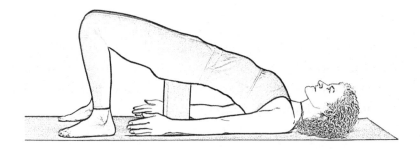

3.  Walk the heels close to the butt, hip distance apart.

4.  Push into the feet and lift the pelvis as high as you can.

5.  Place the block under the sacrum. *Note:* You have three choices of block height. Select the one that will let you hold the pose. Be careful that the yoga block is not in your lumbar spine. The sacrum begins at the top ridge of the buttocks. If you're uncertain, put it closer to the tailbone than the low back.

6.  Keep pressure on the inner heels and mounds of the big toes so the knees don't splay apart.

7.  Draw the upper arms under the torso and toward one another. Push the upper arm bones into the floor and if your arms are long enough, clasp the hands or place your hands against the block.

8.  Keep the chin neutral. Lift the sternum toward the chin; don't tuck the chin toward the sternum.

9.  Stay in the pose for 3–5 minutes or longer.

10. To come out of the pose, push into the feet even more and, using your buttock muscles, lift your pelvis off the block, pull it out from under you, and come back on the floor with control (no flopping or crashing down).

**Modifications**

•   If there is discomfort in the knees, place a block between the thighs and squeeze gently.

**Focused Actions**

- For most students, the inner edge of the foot gets light. Push the soles of the feet into the floor and away from your head. This facilitates a deeper stretch in the upper quadriceps and engages the hamstrings more.

- Draw the top edge of the buttocks away from the lower spine to keep the lumbar from getting compressed.

### *Reclining Bound Angle Pose* (**Supta Baddha Konasana**)

Preview: This is a restorative pose that opens up the pelvic floor muscles, relaxes the abdomen, and increases awareness of the breath in the lower abdomen and perineum.

**Props**

- Bolster
- One to three blankets
- Two blocks
- Strap, fastened in a large loop
- Optional: sandbags
- Optional: yoga eye pillow or soft cloth

**How to Practice**

1. Place the bolster lengthwise toward the back end of the mat and place a folded blanket at the top of the bolster to create a comfortable support for the head and neck.

2. Sit facing away from the bolster in bound angle pose (see page 191), with at least 2–3 inches between you and the front edge of the bolster.

3. Place folded blankets (or yoga blocks can work) under the outer thighs as close to the hip as possible.

4. Bring the looped strap over the torso and down across the sacrum above the tailbone.

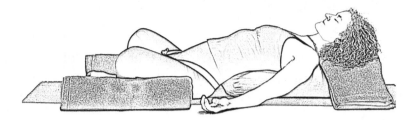

5. Pass it over the inner groin on both sides and around the outer edges of the feet. Pull the strap taut.

6. Lie back onto the bolster. *Note:* After lying back, you may want to momentarily lift the pelvis and draw the buttock flesh away from the lower back to lengthen the lower back.

7. For the next few minutes, focus on deepening your breath and visualizing the inhalation gently opening and stretching the pelvic floor.

8. Remain for 5–20 minutes.

9. To come out of the pose, place the hands under the thighs and bring the knees back together. Slip the feet out of the loop.

10. When you feel ready, bend the knees, turn to your side, and use the hands to push yourself up to sit.

## Modifications

• Place a yoga eye pillow or soft cloth over your eyes to quiet the movement of your eyes. This also blocks stimulating light and deepens relaxation.

• Make sure you are sitting in front of the bolster, not on it. If your lower back feels uncomfortable, then place the bolster on two blocks (at the far end) to angle the back 30° from the floor. If you don't have a bolster, fold three or four firm blankets in narrow rectangles for the same support.

• This pose has more benefits with a strap but can be done without it. The strap lengthens the lower back to take stress off the sacral ligaments, and it holds the feet together, which increases relaxation. The strap also helps traction the lower spine, placing the pelvic floor into a more neutral position, and gently holds the ilia (frontal hip bones) toward each other.

- If you have extra folded blankets or yoga blocks, place them under the forearms with palms of the hands facing up or rest your hands on the belly.

- Place sandbags on the tops of the thighs (be sure there are bolsters or blocks under the thighs before using the sandbags).

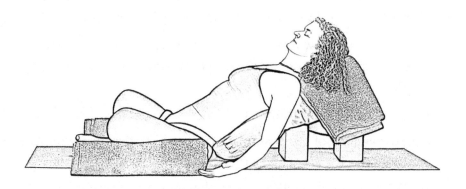

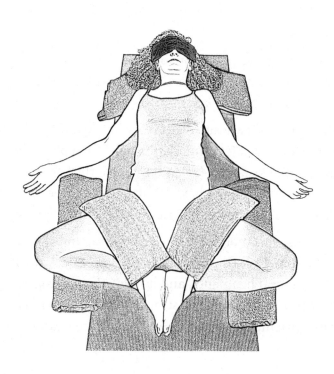

## *Legs on Chair (*Viparita Karani Mudra*)*

Preview: This is a variation of the classical pose where the legs are vertical. This version helps to untuck the pelvis by elevating the buttocks and having the legs supported.

### Props

- Chair
- One or two blankets
- Optional: yoga eye pillow

### How to Practice

1. Sit on a folded blanket with a chair seat facing you. Bend the knees with the feet on the floor.

2. With the hands placed behind the pelvis, lower your back to the floor.

3. Bring the calves up onto the chair seat.

4. Adjust the blanket in the lower back/sacral region so that the pelvis is in neutral and the breath can flow deeply.

5. Let your arms spread away from your body, palms facing up.

6. Stay here, breathing deeply, for 2–20 minutes.

7. Then bring the legs toward the chest and roll to your right side, drawing the knees a little closer to the front body. Take two or three breaths before coming up.

8. To come up, place the left palm in front of the torso. Push into the left hand, allowing the head to come up last.

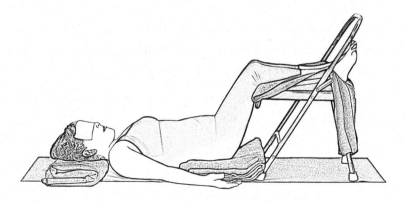

## Modifications

- If you are sensitive to cold, you may want to cover the chair seat with a blanket.

- Place a yoga eye pillow or soft cloth over your eyes to quiet the movement of your eyes. This also blocks stimulating light and deepens relaxation.

- If you have space and hamstring flexibility, you can do this pose with the legs straight up the wall.

- You may be more comfortable with a blanket under the head.

## Focused Actions

- Focus on the breath for the first minute or two: Visualize the pelvic floor softening and releasing on the inhale and the breath moving deeply into the belly.

### *Corpse Pose (*Shavasana*)*

Preview: This pose can be done by itself or as a way to start or end a yoga session. Once you are set up, it is a great way to relax and tune into your breath for 5–15 minutes.

## Props

- Bolster or a few blankets
- Optional: sandbags or a 20–30 pound weight plate
- Optional: yoga eye pillow or scarf to cover the eyes

## How to Practice

1. Sit on the floor with a thickly rolled blanket or bolster under the knees and a blanket ready to go under the head. If you will use an eye pillow, have it nearby.

2. Place the hands behind the hips and lower yourself carefully to the floor.

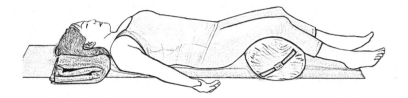

3. Extend the legs. Make sure the bolster is under the knees (centered between the thigh and the shin).

4. Rest the arms, palms up, on the floor about 45° from the torso.

5. Make sure the folded edge of the blanket touches the top of the shoulders, so the blanket under the head is also supporting the neck.

6. Rest the pelvis in a neutral position. *Note:* If the lower back aches, slightly lift the buttocks and use your hands to push the buttock flesh toward the feet. Then bring the pelvis down. Let the legs relax (they will tend to roll out, which is fine).

7. Close the eyes and relax the jaw. Allow the tongue to widen and soften, and, as much as possible, let go of any tension in the body.

8. Stay in this pose for 5–20 minutes.

9. When you are ready to come out of the pose, first focus on the feeling of your body resting on the floor.

10. Then bend the legs, place your feet on the bolster, and roll to your right side, drawing the knees a little closer to the front body. Take two or three breaths before coming up.

11. To come up, place the left palm in front of the torso. Push into the left hand, allowing the head to come up last.

### Modifications

- Bare bones (nothing under you except the mat).
- Place the calves on a chair.

- Place a small support under your Achilles tendons if you have discomfort in the heels or if you want the feeling of extra support.

- Put a blanket over yourself and tuck the blanket under the outside edge of your legs to help keep them slightly more internally rotated. This can help some students access their breath more easily.

**Focused Actions**

- This position will help to deepen your breathing. It can be even more effective if you have some weight on the thighbones. Yoga sandbags are a good option, or you can use a 20–30 pound weight plate.

- Focus on inviting the breath deeper into the belly and encourage its movement toward the pelvic floor. Notice where you feel the movement of the breath. If there are certain places in the body that feel restricted, invite the breath into those places.

- Consider placing an eye pillow, scarf, or towel over the eyes, especially if you are having difficulty relaxing your mind.

## YOGA AND BREATHING
## for Hypotonicity

### *Relaxation Pose with Weight* (Shavasana)

Preview: This setup is the same as for *shavasana* (relaxation pose) on page 164. Here, the focus is on inviting the breath to go deeper and more fully into the lower torso. Remember, deep breathing helps the pelvic floor stretch on the inhale and contract on the exhale. The stretch should not happen because you are manipulating the muscles; the positive effect on the pelvic floor happens as a result of better breathing.

**Props**

- Blankets: one folded for under the head, one folded to put across your thighs
- Bolster or rolled blanket for under the knees
- Strap if you have issues with sacral instability
- Two yoga sandbags, 8–10 pounds each. *Note:* If you use a weight plate (20–30 pounds) instead, use an extra yoga mat to secure the plate on top of your legs
- Optional:
  - Blanket to cover yourself
  - Rolled blanket under the Achilles tendon
  - Yoga eye pillow or scarf to place over the eyes

**How to Practice**

1. Place your mat on the floor (a firm surface is crucial) with the blanket for your head support in place and ready for when you lie down.

2. Sit on your mat with a bolster or blanket under your knees. (If you are using a belt, place the belt on the mid thigh so that the thighs are a little less externally rotated.)

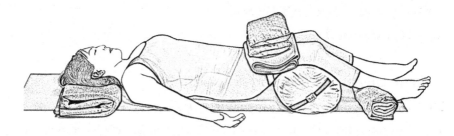

3.  If you are using sandbags, place them directly on your thighs. *Note:* The sandbags can be cold so you might want to put a folded mat or blanket across your thighs. If you tend to get cold, cover your body.

4.  Lie down on your back with legs extended and arms at your sides, about 6 inches away from the body with the palms up.

5.  Let the legs relax. Close the eyes.

6.  Shift the focus of your attention to the sensations in the belly and lower back; the movement of the breath will become less pronounced in the chest.

7.  Imagine your body releasing toward the ground.

8.  From the soles of the feet to the crown of the head, consciously release every body part, limb, organ, and cell.

9.  Relax the face. Let the eyes drop deep into the sockets. Invite the breath to come into the pelvic floor. A general guideline is to stay in *shavasana* 5 minutes for every 30 minutes of your practice.

10. To exit the pose, begin to deepen the breath, bringing gentle movement and awareness back to the body, wiggling the fingers and toes.

11. Roll to the right side and rest there for a moment. With an inhalation, gently press the left hand into the floor to come into a comfortable seated position.

### Shavasana with Elevated Pelvis and Legs on Chair

Preview: Follow instructions for *shavasana*, page 199, put a blanket or two under your pelvis, and place the calves on the seat of a folding chair to elevate the legs. You may want to put a blanket on the chair seat to keep your legs warm. This is a great variation if you are dealing with a prolapsed organ. It helps to take the weight off the pelvic floor while you are relaxing.

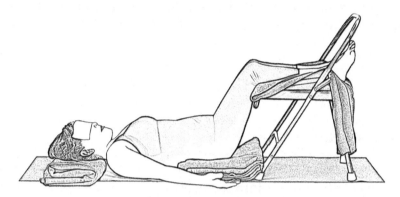

## Poses for Hypotonicity

Practice these specific yoga postures and techniques with the goal of strengthening the muscles of the pelvic floor, which was shown in the UCSF study to improve urinary incontinence.[2] Strengthening the pelvic floor muscles can also help with some forms of bladder, uterine, and rectal prolapse. Remember that if you have any tightness or pain in your pelvic floor muscles, you should practice the poses for hypertonicity, not hypotonicity, as you cannot strengthen muscles that are already contracted. When the pelvic floor muscles start to release, stretch, and soften, you can begin to introduce some of these poses that are more for stability and strength.

All of these poses can be done as a group or on their own.

### *Mountain Pose (*Tadasana*) with Block between Inner Legs*

Preview: This is an extremely important pose because it can improve your general standing position in life. It is a template for all of the standing poses. Holding a yoga block between the upper thighs highlights the connection between the feet, legs, and pelvic floor. This teaches the neutral position of the spine (normal curvature; no flat back) and pelvis, so that pelvic floor muscle function is maximized. This pose takes work—don't think of it as just standing around!

**Props**

- Yoga block

**How to Practice**

1. Stand with the weight balanced evenly on both feet. Shift a little more weight into the heels.

2. Place the yoga block (narrowest side) between the upper inner thighs.

3. Push the femurs back and ensure the pelvis is in neutral so that the center of the perineum is parallel to the floor and in line with the crown of the head. *Note:* You might feel like you are sticking your tail out more than you are used to. This could be a good sign if you tend to be a mothertucker.

4. Push down actively through the heels and the balls of the feet. This awakens the energy line that runs from the inner arch up the inseam of the leg into the perineum. It should feel like the block is being lifted toward the perineum.

5. Lift the crown of the head away from the perineum.

6. Remain in this pose for 1–5 minutes.

## Modifications

- Practice the pose with the block between the calves for slightly different effects. Gently hug the brick with your lower legs and imagine the action is coming from your outer calves.

## Focused Actions

- Be mindful not to let your tailbone tuck under you, and don't allow the thighbones to come forward and roll out.

- Rotate the thighs inward slightly (the block rolls behind you). This action creates space on each side of the tailbone and spreads the sitting bones. This also sets the pelvis up to be in neutral, which enables the pubic bone to support the bladder.

- To deepen your awareness of subtle sensation, practice in succession gently lifting the anal sphincter, then the urethral sphincter, squeezing the vaginal walls, and lifting the perineum. This teaches the body and brain that these are four different and distinct actions and areas. They should all feel slightly different.

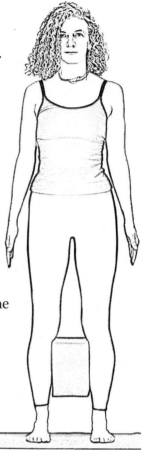

## *Intense Side Stretch Pose* (**Parshvottanasana**)

Preview: This pose works the legs and helps you to feel the connection of the feet, the legs, and the pelvic floor.

## Props

- Two yoga blocks
- Optional: a chair if the hamstrings are very tight

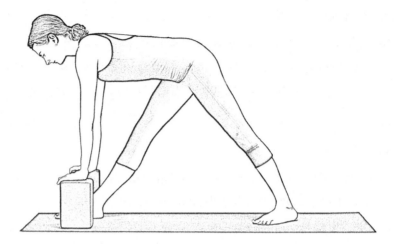

**How to Practice**

1. Stand in tadasana at the front edge of the mat with a yoga block just outside the outer edge of each foot.

2. Place the hands on the hips. Step the left leg back 2.5–3 feet, keeping the front hip points facing the same direction.

3. While pushing down into the inner and outer heels, contract the quadriceps to keep the kneecaps lifted and legs straight.

4. Align the perineum under the crown of the head.

5. Hinging from the hips and keeping the head in line with the torso, lengthen the front of the spine forward over the front (right) leg. Stop when the torso is parallel to the floor or when the back begins to round, whichever happens first.

6. Lightly place the fingertips on the blocks.

7. Extend the outer heel of the back leg toward the floor. Lift the inner arch of the foot toward the perineum.

8. Keep the inner heel of the front foot pressing firmly into the floor. Press the base of the big toe down. Lift the inner groin of the right leg deep into the perineum.

9. Hold this pose for 30–60 seconds.

10. To come out of the pose, inhale and hinge the torso up, starting from the base of the spine. Repeat on the other side.

## Modifications

- If this pose feels unstable, take the right foot an inch to the right so that the feet are wider from left to right.

- If you are still having difficulty keeping your balance in this pose, you can use the wall to stabilize through the back heel or you can stand so that you are oriented with your shoulder and hip adjacent to the wall.

- Additionally, you can place your hands on a chair instead of blocks, but put the chair on your yoga mat so that it doesn't slip.

## Focused Actions

- While working the feet and legs in this pose, imagine an energy line from the inner arches of the feet to the perineum. The more you can push down into the heels, the more lift you get in the pelvic floor.

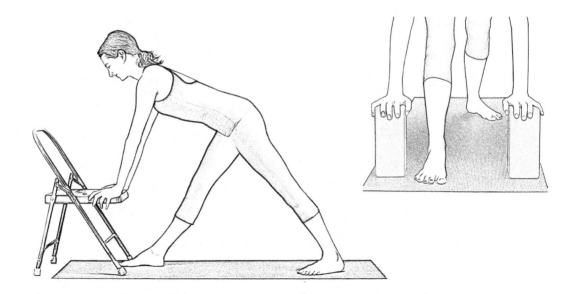

### *Chair Pose (*Utkatasana*)*

Preview: This pose strengthens the hamstrings and buttocks. It is useful as an exercise for training the pelvic floor to remain stable in transitions between sitting and standing. This posture can be practiced dynamically. When practiced with pelvic awareness, it helps to stretch the pelvic floor muscles as you move into the pose, and to engage the pelvic floor muscles to stabilize the trunk and pelvis while in the pose. It also helps the pelvic floor muscles when moving out of the pose into mountain pose.

#### Props

- Optional: yoga block for between the thighs, as in mountain pose

#### How to Practice

1. Start in mountain pose (*tadasana*) with the hands on the hips. Place a block between the upper thighs on the narrowest width.

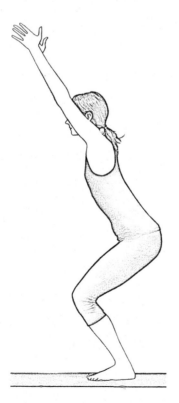 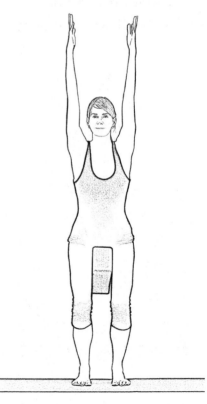

2. Bend the knees, making sure the kneecaps track straight ahead.

3. Move the buttocks back as if you were going to sit in a chair. Be vigilant about not tucking the pelvis.

4. As the knees bend, keep the weight more in the heels. Push into the inner and outer heels. Lift the inseam of the thighs toward the perineum as if you were lifting the block to the perineum.

5. Remain in this pose for 30 seconds, working up to 1 minute. For a more challenging variation, extend the arms up rather than keeping the hands on the hips.

6. To come out of the pose, on an exhalation, push into the heels and straighten the legs while lifting the pelvic floor. Notice how the sitting bones come together as the legs straighten.

## Modifications

- If free standing is not possible due to weakness in the legs, stand in front of your kitchen sink (or an equally stable structure) and hold the edge for support while bending and straightening the legs. Coordinate movement and breathing.

- If you feel the sitting bones moving toward each other when going into the pose, this indicates that the pelvis is tucking.

## Focused Actions

- Work to keep the body's weight more in the heels. Keep the spine perpendicular to the floor. Minimize how much the upper body tips forward.

- Keep the inner thighs rolling in slightly with the knees pointing straight ahead. Beware of the tendency for the knees to collapse in. This makes the ankles and inner arches collapse and that puts extra strain on the pelvic floor. Also, don't let the knees splay out, which places too much weight on the outer edges of the feet.

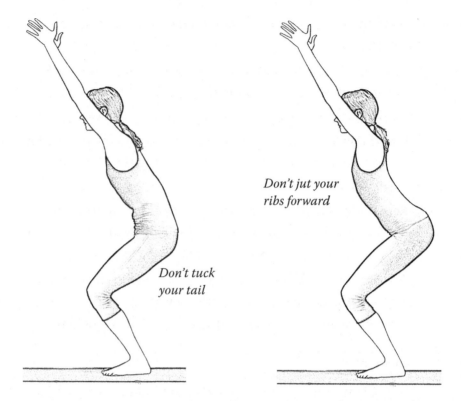

*Don't jut your ribs forward*

*Don't tuck your tail*

- Visualize your anatomy as you move in and out of the pose. As the knees bend into the pose, the sitting bones move apart from each other and the pelvic floor stretches. As the knees straighten moving out of the pose, the sitting bones draw toward each other and the pelvic floor gently engages and lifts. This pose can be practiced dynamically, by slightly bending and straightening the legs in coordination with the inhale and the exhale, respectively.

### Goddess Pose

Preview: Goddess pose strengthens the lower body, activates the gluteus muscles, and encourages the breath into the abdomen. Goddess pose is excellent for cultivating pelvic floor muscle awareness, and it links the action of the feet, inner legs, and pelvic floor. Similar to chair pose, goddess pose can be done dynamically with the breath (inhale down, exhale up) or statically.

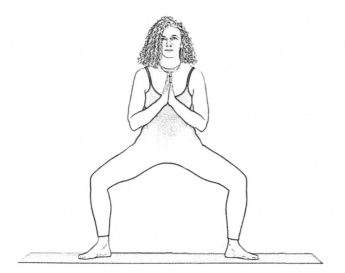

## How to Practice

1. Start from mountain pose (*tadasana*).

2. Step the feet 2–2.5 feet apart. Turn the feet out slightly with hands on the hips and the pelvis in neutral.

3. Keeping the perineum parallel to the floor and the spine as upright as possible, slowly bend the knees so that the kneecaps face away from each other and the thighs are close to parallel with the floor. Bring palms together in front of the chest.

4. Push down into the inner heels and lift up through the inner thighs to the perineum. Squeeze the inner heels toward one another while keeping the pelvis in neutral.

5. Stay 10–30 seconds or move dynamically with the breath for 30 seconds to 1 minute.

6. To come out, strongly push into the heels, straighten the legs, and bring the feet together.

## Modifications

• Hold onto something solid (like the kitchen sink).

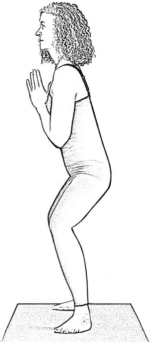

*Pelvis neutral; be careful not to tuck your pelvis as shown here.*

### Focused Actions

- To help engage and strengthen the pelvic floor muscles, pull the inner heels toward each other while maintaining foot position. This might help you feel how the action of the feet, inner leg, and perineum connect and support each other.

- Don't let your tailbone tuck under you or allow the thighbones or knees to roll in.

- This pose can be done with different types of pelvic floor contractions: dynamic goddess, with quick, pulsating lifts, or static goddess, with sustained contraction and pelvic lift.

### *Warrior 2 (*Virabhadrasana 2)

Preview: Standing poses help you find the connection between the feet, legs, and pelvic floor. The grounding of the feet and external rotation of the thighbones contract the pelvic floor muscles and stabilize the torso.

### How to Practice

1. Start in mountain pose. Separate the feet 3–3.5 feet, more if you have long legs.

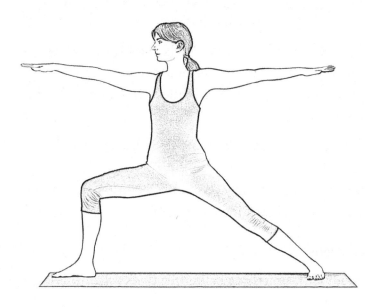

2.  Turn the left foot in about 45°.

3.  Turn the right foot and leg out 90°.

4.  Align the heel of the right foot with the heel of the left.

5.  Place the hands on the hips. Push weight into the front heel and the back foot.

6.  Gently squeeze the heels toward each other on the mat as if there were a spring between them.

7.  While actively pushing the heels down, strongly contract the quadriceps muscles to stabilize the knee joints.

8.  Rotate the thighbones externally. *Note:* External rotation of the legs will help engage the pelvic floor muscles and draw the sitting bones together.

9.  Raise the arms parallel to the floor and reach them away from each other.

10. Bend the right knee so that the shin is perpendicular to the floor. *Note:* The right knee should be aligned directly over the right ankle. The right thigh should be as close to parallel with the ground as possible.

11. Press down through the inner and outer edges of the back foot. Keep the back leg straight and externally rotated with the kneecap lifted. *Note:* There should be more weight in the back leg than the front leg.

12. Keep the torso perpendicular to the floor. Align the crown of the head over the perineum; do not lean toward the front leg.

13. Draw the pubic bone toward the navel. Lengthen the top buttock flesh away from the lumbar spine.

14. Turn the head to gaze out across the tip of the right middle finger.

15. Hold this pose for up to 1 minute.

16. To release, inhale as you press down through the back foot and straighten the front leg. Lower the arms.

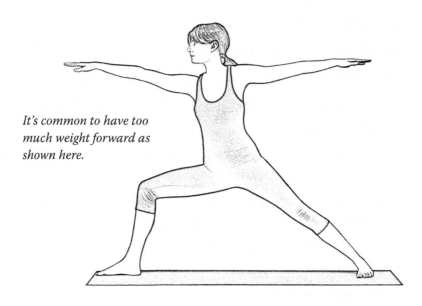

*It's common to have too much weight forward as shown here.*

17. Turn to the left, reversing the position of the feet.

18. Repeat for the same length of time on the opposite side.

## Modifications

- If you find your weight falling into the front leg, put your back heel against the wall to help keep your focus there.

- If balance is a challenge in this pose, stand with your back at a wall. The wall can be used as a support for the head and upper body.

## Focused Actions

- The more you can externally rotate your thighbones, the more the pelvic floor muscles engage, especially the second layer.

- It is common to have too much weight forward. Remember to lift through the crown of the head.

### *Triangle Pose (*Trikonasana*)*

Preview: This pose encourages active engagement of the pelvic floor muscles, especially through the positioning, external rotation, and work of the legs.

#### Props

- Yoga block or chair

#### How to Practice

1. Start at the front of your mat in mountain pose.

2. With the block or chair at your right outer shin, step your left foot back 3–3½ feet, more if you have long legs.

3. Turn your left foot in about 45° and turn the right foot and leg out 90°. Align the heel of the right foot with the heel of the left.

4. Place the hands on the hips and push more weight into the heels. Strongly squeeze the heels toward each other and draw your energy up the inner leg and into the perineum.

5. While actively pushing the heels down, strongly contract the quadriceps muscles to stabilize the knee joints and rotate the thighbones externally. *Note:* External rotation of the legs will help engage your pelvic floor muscles and draw the sitting bones together.

6. Raise the arms parallel to the floor and reach them away from each other.

7. Anchoring the inner and outer heel of the left foot, extend the torso to the right, directly over the plane of the right leg. *Note:* Side bend from the hip joint, not the waist.

8. Place your right hand on the support. Stretch the left arm toward the ceiling.

9. Push the inner heel of your right foot into the ground as you work to externally rotate the right thigh. Bring the right-leg sitting bone toward the perineum.

10. Keep the head in a neutral position, in line with the spine.

11. Remain in this pose for 1 minute.

12. To come out of the pose, stand up on an inhale, strongly pressing the back heel into the floor.

13. Reverse the feet and repeat the pose for the same length of time on the other side.

## Modifications

- If you find your weight falling into the front leg, put your back heel against the wall to help keep your focus there, or take more height under your hand, such as two stacked blocks or the sandbag.

- If balance is a challenge in this pose, stand with your back to a wall and put your yoga block between your front outer shin and the wall.

## Focused Actions

- The more you can externally rotate your thighbones, the more the pelvic floor muscles engage, especially the second layer.

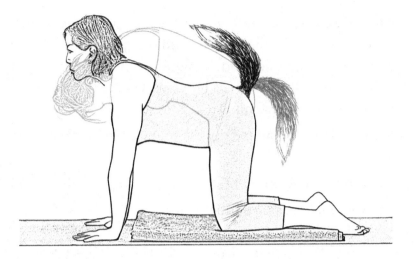

## *Tabletop, Cat-Cow*

Preview: This pose is useful for feeling the muscles of the pelvic floor, especially layers one and three. This pose is highly recommended for a prolapsed uterus, bladder, or rectum. You will experience tucking and untucking the pelvis; this shortens and lengthens the pelvic floor muscles from pubic bone to tailbone. When doing cat-cow, link movement and breath. This is an exaggeration of what happens in normal breathing with regard to the movement of the pelvis.

### Props

- Optional: a blanket to pad the knees

### How to Practice

1. Tabletop: Come onto the hands and knees with the pelvis in neutral, hands directly under the shoulder joints, and knees directly below the hip joints, with tops of feet flat on the floor.

2. Cow: On the inhale, lift the head and the tailbone toward the ceiling, arching the back. Lengthen the front abdominal muscles. *Note:* When head and tail are up, the pelvic floor is lengthening.

3. Cat: On the exhale, round the spine up toward the ceiling. Draw the sides of the navel toward the spine. Move the head and tail toward one another, rounding the back and tucking the pelvis. *Note:* When the head and tail are tucked, the pelvic floor is shortening.

4. Move between cow and cat 3–5 rounds, following the breath.

5. Return to tabletop.

6. Engage and release your perineum (quick flicks) 5–6 times, rest for a few breaths. Then practice longer holds (5–10 seconds), without holding the breath. Pause between each longer hold.

> "Quick flicks" are just what they sound like, pulsating the pelvic floor muscles quickly for one second in succession.

**Modifications**

- If bearing weight on the wrists is not possible, you can do this with your forearms on blocks or, if comfortable, curl your hands into fists and rest on the knuckles with wrists in neutral.

**Focused Actions**

- Practice both quick lifts (pulsations) and more sustained holds without holding the breath.

### Plank Pose

Preview: This is one of the best poses to build abdominal and pelvic floor strength. This is recommended for those with a prolapsed organ. When practicing plank, the pelvic organs are resting forward of the pelvic floor muscles, not on them. It can take time to build the strength to hold the pose for more than a breath or two. Be gentle with yourself while building up stamina.

**Props**

- Optional: yoga wedges if you need wrist support

**How to Practice**

1. Begin on the hands and knees, with the shoulders directly over the wrists.

2. Spread the fingers and press down through the root of the index fingers. *Note:* Do not let the breastbone collapse toward the ground; draw the abdominal muscles toward the spine.

3. Keep the neck in a neutral position by holding the gaze between the hands.

4. Tuck the toes under and step back, one foot at a time. Bring the body and head into one straight line.

5. Keep the thighs lifted and abs engaged so the hips don't sink. If the buttocks are high in the air (be glad you noticed!), realign the body so the shoulders are directly over the wrists.

6. Draw the pelvic floor muscles toward the head; contract the abdominal muscles.

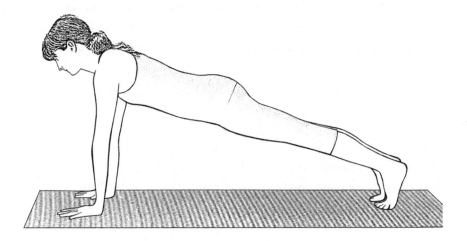

7.  Broaden across the upper back, creating space between the shoulder blades; widen the collarbones.

8.  Press the fronts of the thighs (quadriceps) up toward the ceiling. Keep the lower back in a neutral position. In other words, don't tuck or overarch the back!

9.  Hold for 3–5 breaths.

10. To come out, bend the knees and take the buttocks back toward the heels for child's pose.

## Modifications

- Use yoga wedges if you need wrist support, or come on to your forearms.

- If you don't feel strong enough to support the full body weight, lower the knees to the floor.

- To deepen the pose, try lifting one leg at a time. Hold the lifted leg for 3–5 breaths. Repeat with the opposite leg for the same amount of time.

## Focused Actions

- When you focus on lifting the pelvic floor, think about starting the action from the perineum. Ideally, you will feel all of your abdominal muscles contact more. Firm the buttocks, but not so much that you are going into posterior tilt—no tucking!

### *Thunderbolt (*Vajrasana*)*[3]

Preview: This pose increases the flexibility of the ankles, knees, and thighs. If done with a focus on the pelvic floor, the work of the lower legs directly engages the perineum and lifts the spine. This is one of the best "seated" poses for connecting the feet with the pelvic floor.

## Props

- Bolster

- One to three blankets

**How to Practice**

1. Kneel on the floor with the thighs together, knees in line with hips, toes untucked, and heels in line with the sitting bones. Put a thinly folded blanket under just the knees; this helps put more weight in the feet. *Note:* You may want a blanket on the mat to pad the knees, shins, and ankles.

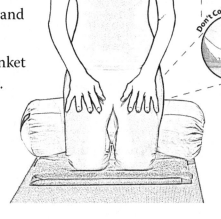

2. Place a bolster or thickly folded blanket between the heels and the buttocks.

3. Bring the buttocks back onto the heels. *Note:* In this transition from kneeling to sitting on the heels, strongly lift the tailbone and sitting bones to maintain a neutral pelvis. Keep the weight of the torso directly over the sitting bones. Do not tuck your tail under as you sit down. If this happens, add more height between the buttocks and heels. During the transition, the heels will try to splay away from each other, so actively hug the outer heels, outer ankles, and outer calves toward the midline.

4. Rest the hands on the tops of the thighs near the knees, with the palms down. The elbows should be slightly bent.

5. To engage the pelvic floor, press the top of the feet, front of the ankles, and front of the shin bones down. Continue to hug the outer heels, outer ankles, and outer calves toward the midline. This brings awareness to the perineum and lifts it.

6. Remain in this pose for 1–5 minutes.

**Modifications**

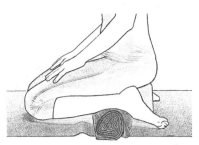

- If this pose causes too much discomfort in the fronts of the ankles, place a rolled blanket between the floor and the front of the ankle so the feet hang off the blanket roll. Or place an extra blanket to make a ledge for the lower leg, knee to ankle, to rest on and allow the feet to hang off. The ledge reduces the angle of plantar flexion required to assume this pose.

- If your knees hurt, try putting a blanket or rolled up washcloth behind them. Note that some discomfort when the quads and ankles stretch is normal, as is some pressure in the knees. But a sharp pain in the knees shouldn't be tolerated.

**Focused Actions**

- To help cultivate more awareness of the pelvic floor, place a rolled yoga strap under the perineum.

- When in this pose, you can also work on sustained holds of the pelvic floor muscles with the described action in the lower leg as well as quick flick one second lifting pulsations of the pelvic muscles.

- For a counter stretch to the feet you can also switch the toes to be tucked and sit on the heels.

## *Squat Pose* (Malasana)

CAUTION: **Do not do this pose if you have any knowledge or suspicion of a prolapse. Squatting puts pressure into the pelvis, and if not done carefully and with correct alignment, your condition could worsen. If you know of or suspect a prolapse, do the supine version.**

Preview: This pose increases the sensation in and awareness of your pelvic floor muscles. It is performed squatting on the floor with support under the heels. If the knees or back are problematic, practice with a blanket or mat behind the knees. If the upright position is not possible, the pose can be done on the floor on your back by drawing the knees in toward the chest. The flexion of the hips in this pose prevents the buttocks from working. Usually the pelvic floor can be contracted at will in this position without other muscles substituting or taking over.

### How to Practice

1. Stand in mountain pose with a rolled up blanket or yoga mat under the heels, feet about hip distance apart. *Note:* Even if you can keep the heels fully on the floor in this pose, use the support under them so that the pelvis can be neutral.

2. Slowly bend your knees, dropping the weight into the heels, as though you were going to sit down in a chair.

3. Come into a squat; maintain equal weight in the inner and outer heels. Allow the knees to be a bit wider than the torso.

4. Bring the palms together and press the elbows out against the inner thighs. At the same time, resist the elbows with the knees.

5. Remain in this pose for 30 seconds to 2 minutes.

6.  To come out of the pose, put the hands on the floor and slowly lift the pelvis up toward the ceiling, coming into a standing forward bend. Take a few breaths before standing fully upright. Hinge from the hips to come up.

**Modifications**

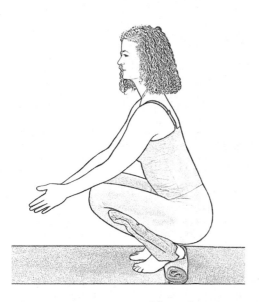

- If your knees bother you while squatting, put a thinly folded blanket behind them as you go down.

- If you feel dizzy coming out of this pose, rise very slowly on an inhalation. Alternatively, come onto the hands and knees before coming up and out of the pose.

- If you feel unsteady in this pose, you can do it with a chair in front of you to help with balance. To come out of the pose, push your hands on the chair seat.

- If you have a rounder belly so that it's uncomfortable to have the hands folded together in front of the chest, let the hands lightly hold the front of the knees.

**Focused Actions**

- Visualize the diamond shape of the bony structure of the pelvic floor while you lift the perineum up toward the crown of the head.

- Isolate the action of the pelvic floor muscles without using the buttocks.

- When pressing the elbows out into the legs and legs into the elbows, lift the perineum toward the crown of the head. You may work on quick flicks or sustained holds of the pelvic floor muscles.

- You can alternate hand-to-knee position by putting the hands on the outsides of the knees and pressing out with the knees to encourage a subtle action of contrast.

### *Bound Angle Pose (*Baddha Konasana*)*

Preview: This pose should be practiced seated on either the edge of several firm stacked blankets or a block. If your knees are still higher than your hip crease, sit on a bolster in front of a wall, and lean into the wall. This allows the knees to drop below the level of the hip joints, which stretches the inner thighs and layer two of the pelvic floor when the pelvis is in neutral. This pose can be used to contract and strengthen the pelvic floor muscles, or it can be done passively to stretch the pelvic floor.

### Props

- Two to three blankets or one blanket and one bolster
- Two blocks, placed close behind you

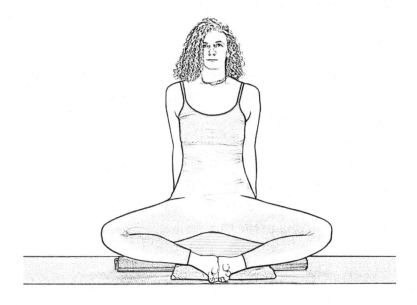

**How to Practice**

1.  Sit in staff pose (page 127) with a support that allows the pelvis to be in neutral. The perineum should be parallel to the floor and lined up with the crown of the head. The energetic tail should be behind you, as described in the earlier section about neutral pelvis (page 99).

2.  Bend the knees to join the soles of the feet together. Keep the heels (especially outer heels) together and let the knees drop outward. Bring the feet as close to the pelvis as is comfortable.

3.  Place your hands on the blocks and push down to lengthen the spine up.

4.  Firmly push the heels into each other and lengthen the inner thighs toward the inner knees. Make sure to keep the outer edges of the feet firmly together. Allow the toes to come away from each other.

5.  Stay in this pose for 3–5 minutes, alternating actively pressing into the heels and relaxing.

6.  To come out of the pose, use the hands to push the outer knees together, and then extend the legs in front of you.

**Modifications**

*   If there is any discomfort in your knees, place a rolled up washcloth behind each knee to create space.

*   A variation of the pose that alleviates minor knee pain: Roll up a hand towel and slide the rolled towel under the heels, toes remain touching the floor so that the ankles remain neutral (not overstretched on the outer ankle). This can also be done with a sandbag. This variation also maximizes external rotation of the thighbones.

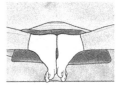

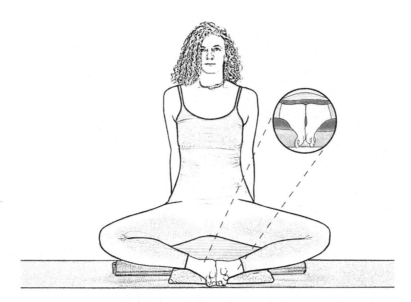

## Focused Actions

- Feel the difference in your pelvic floor when actively pushing the heels together and actively lengthening the inner legs away from each other, compared with sitting passively.

- When doing this pose actively, notice that the sitting bones may work differently on the two sides. Work to make the pelvic floor engage more evenly.

### *Supported Bridge Pose (*Setu Bandhasana Sarvanghasana*)*

Preview: This pose takes the weight of the organs off the pelvic floor. For hypotonicity, this pose is done with a block under the sacrum to bring awareness to the nuances of activating the pelvic floor and to link the heels with the legs and the pelvic floor. See "Smart Ass, Dumb Ass" on page 177 for a more diagnostic version of the pose.

### Props

- Yoga block

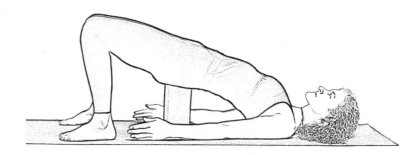

**How to Practice**

1.  Lie on your back on the floor with the yoga block at hand.

2.  Bend the knees 90°, bringing the heels close to the buttocks and keeping the feet hip distance apart.

3.  Keeping knees in line with hips, pushing into the heels, lift the pelvis as high as you can.

4.  Place the block underneath the sacrum. *Note:* The height of the block will depend on how high you can lift the pelvis.

5.  Roll the arms out with the palms up. Press the upper arms into the floor to keep the chest lifting toward the chin. Keep the chin neutral; do not tuck the chin to the sternum.

6.  Strongly press the inner and outer heels into the ground. Engage the pelvic floor.

7.  Stay in the pose for 1–3 minutes.

8.  To come out of the pose, press into the heels and lift the pelvis off the block. Put the block to the side. Come down slowly, lengthening the lower back to rest the back on the floor.

**Modifications**

•   If the knees splay out, or if you have any discomfort in the knee, place a yoga block between the thighs to keep them internally rotated.

•   If the feet splay out (duck feet), place a yoga block between the ankles.

**Focused Actions**

- Contract the pelvic floor for as long as you can (up to 10 seconds), then rest. Repeat this at least three times.

- To vary the work, relax the legs and buttocks and engage the pelvic floor to do quick flicks and more sustained holds.

## *Half Locust Pose* (Ardha Shalabhasana)

Preview: Some students with weak and hypotonic pelvic floors have non-working butts (or should I say unemployed). This can occur in the whole buttocks or on one side more than the other, which is common. This pose helps balance the buttock muscles and the pelvic floor muscles.

**Props**

- Blanket to pad the hip bones
- Blanket to support the forehead

**How to Practice**

1. Spread a blanket across the mat to provide padding for the pelvis; place another blanket for under your forehead.

2. Lie on the belly with the arms behind your torso, forehead on the blanket. Press your fingertips into the right mid buttock. Turn the thighbones inward to create space around the tailbone.

3. On an exhale lift the perineum and gently draw the abdomen away from the floor at the same time. Raise the

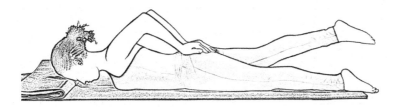

right leg up. Draw the tops of the buttocks toward the bottoms of the buttocks.

4. Keep the leg raised for 30–60 seconds, remembering to breathe, while maintaining the lift in the perineum and abdomen. Push into your buttocks to make sure it is very firm.

5. Lower the leg on an exhalation.

6. Take a few breaths and repeat on the left side. Notice if one side does not engage and firm as well as the other. If you notice this do a few extra repetitions on your weaker side.

7. Then lift the legs together and compare the two sides. Hold for 30 seconds and slowly lower the legs and then relax your abdomen and pelvic floor.

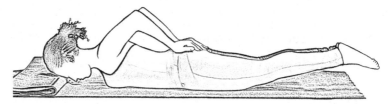

### Modifications

• If your lower back compresses, make sure you are engaging the abdominal muscles. Also, don't lift the leg so high.

• Often the two buttocks don't work to the same capacity. This can contribute to imbalance in the pelvic floor muscles. If you notice this, practice on the weaker side a few extra times.

• A fun variation to add a chest opener is to clasp the hands behind the back while lifting the legs.

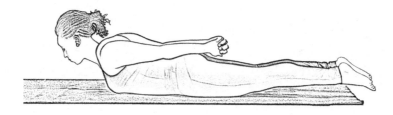

**Focused Actions**

- Ensure that the pelvic floor is lifting, not pushing down. Practice engaging the pelvic floor and the abdominal muscles at the same time.

### *Reclining Bound Angle Pose (*Supta Baddha Konasana*)*

Preview: This is a restorative pose that opens up the pelvic floor muscles, relaxes the abdomen, and increases awareness of the breath in the lower abdomen and perineum.

**Props**

- Bolster
- One to three blankets
- Two blocks
- Strap, fastened into a loop
- Optional: sandbags for the thighs
- Optional: eye bag

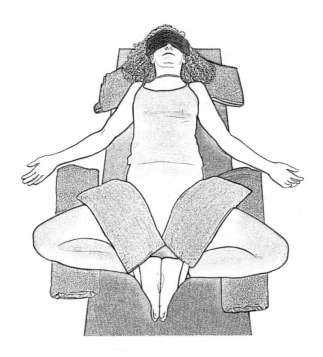

**How to Practice**

1. Place the bolster lengthwise toward the back end of the mat. Place a folded blanket at the top of the bolster to create a comfortable support for the head and neck.

2. Sit facing away from the bolster with at least 2–3 inches between you and the front edge of the bolster.

3. Place folded blankets (or yoga blocks) under the outer thighs as close to the hip as possible.

4. Pulling the looped strap over the head, bring it behind the back at the level of the sacrum (above the tailbone, not the waist). Place the other end of the looped strap around the tops of the feet. Make the strap taught.

5. Lie back onto the bolster. After lying back, you may want to momentarily lift the pelvis and draw the buttock flesh away from the lower back to lengthen the lower back.

6. For the first minute, focus on deepening the breath and visualizing the breath gently opening the pelvic floor on the inhale.

7. Remain in the pose for 5–20 minutes.

8. To come out, place the hands under the thighs and bring the knees back together; slip the feet out of the loop.

9. When you feel ready, bend the knees, turn to the right side, and use the left hand to slowly push yourself up.

**Modifications**

- Place a yoga eye pillow, scarf, or soft cloth over the eyes. This will quiet eye movements and allow for deeper relaxation.

- Make sure you are sitting in front of the bolster, not on it. If the lower back feels uncomfortable, place two blocks under the bolster (at the far end) to angle the back 30° from the floor. If you don't have a bolster, you can fold three or four firm blankets into a narrow rectangle for the same support.

- This pose has more benefits with a strap, but can be done without it. The strap lengthens the lower back to take stress off the sacral ligaments. The strap also holds the feet together, which increases relaxation. It also helps traction the lower spine, placing the pelvic floor into a more neutral position.

- Take support (extra blankets or blocks) under the forearms. Hands can stay at your sides or rest on the belly.

- If you have sandbags, place them on the tops of the thighs. However, it is important that you never put weight on the thighs without having support under them first.

### Corpse Pose (Shavasana)

Preview: This pose can be done by itself or as a way to start or end a yoga session. Once you are set up, it is a great way to relax and tune into your breath for 5–15 minutes.

#### Props

- Bolster or a few blankets for under the knees
- Blanket for under the head
- Yoga eye pillow or scarf to cover the eyes

#### How to Practice

1. Sit on the floor with a rolled blanket or bolster under the knees. Have a blanket ready to support the head. If you have an eye pillow, place it nearby.

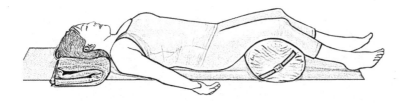

2.　Place the hands behind the hips and lower yourself carefully to the floor. Extend the legs. Make sure the bolster is under the knees, centered between the thigh and the shin. Let the arms rest on the floor about 45° from the torso, with palms facing up. Make sure that the edge of the blanket under the head touches the top of the shoulders to support the neck as well as the head.

3.　Have the pelvis in an anatomically neutral position. *Note:* If the lower back aches, lift the buttocks slightly and use the hands to push the buttock flesh toward the feet, then bring the pelvis back down to the floor.

4.　Let the legs relax; they will tend to roll out due to gravity.

5.　Close the eyes, relax the jaw, and allow the tongue to widen and soften. Scan the body and let go of any tension.

6.　Stay in this pose for 5–20 minutes.

7.　When you're ready to come out of the pose, take a few moments and focus on the sensations of the back of the body resting on the floor.

8.　Bend the legs and place the feet on the bolster.

9.　Roll to the right side, drawing the knees a little closer to the front body. Take two or three breaths before coming up. Then place the left palm on the floor beside you and push into the left hand as you come up. Let the head come up last.

### Modifications

•　If your low back tends to ache, place the calves on a chair or put a belt around the thighs so they don't roll out so much.

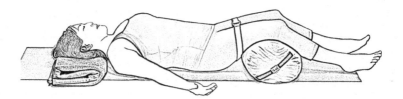

- You can also place a small support under your Achilles tendons if you have discomfort in the heels or if you want extra support.

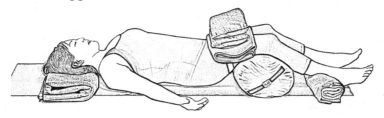

- You can put a blanket over yourself and tuck the blanket under the outside edge of your legs to help keep them slightly more internally rotated.

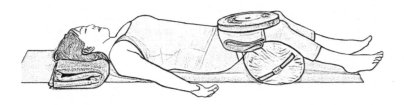

- If you are having difficulty relaxing your mind, consider placing an eye pillow or towel over your eyes to quiet eye movements.

**Focused Actions**

- This position will help to deepen and lengthen your inhales and exhales. It is even more effective if you have some weight, such as sandbags made especially as yoga props, on the thighbones.
- Focus on inviting the breath to come deeper in the belly and toward the pelvic floor. Notice where you feel the movement caused by this deeper breathing and if there are places in the body that feel restricted. Invite your breath into those places.

### Legs Up the Wall Pose *(Viparita Karani Variation)*

Preview: This posture removes the weight of gravity from the pelvic floor and induces a generally relaxed state.

#### Props

- Two blankets

#### How to Practice

1. Pad your mat with a blanket. Use a second blanket under the head.

2. Sit sideways to a wall with one hip touching the wall.

3. Bend the knees, swivel the hips, and extend the legs up the wall so that you land in an L shape with the back flat on the floor.

4. Remain in the pose for 2–10 minutes.

5. To come out of the pose, bend the knees, roll to one side, and use the arms to push yourself up to sitting.

#### Modifications

- If your hamstring muscles are very tight, move your pelvis away from the wall a bit. Or your calves can be supported on a chair.

- Cover yourself with a blanket if you tend to get cold.

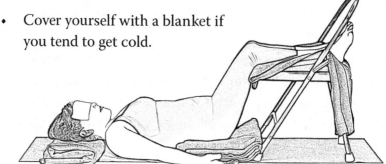

## Poses to Be a Smart Ass: Yoga for the Gluteal Muscles

Here's a short practice for awareness and strengthening of the gluteus muscles. Before doing this practice, you may want to stretch your glutes and hamstrings with reclining big toe pose (page 99) and downward facing dog pose (page 164).

### *Half Bridge Pose* (Setu Bandhasana Sarvanghasana)

Preview: The difference between this version and the ones taught in the two pelvic sequences is that the heels are worked asymmetrically to train the glutes to work symmetrically. This helps if you have left-right disparity; do a few extra repetitions and holds on your weaker side.

**How to Practice**

1.  Lie on your back on the floor.
2.  Bend the knees 90°, heels close to the buttocks, feet hip distance apart.
3.  Have the arms alongside the body.
4.  Bring the right thigh with knee still bent toward the chest. If you need to, hold the thigh with the right hand.
5.  Press the left heel into the floor. Lift the ball of the foot.

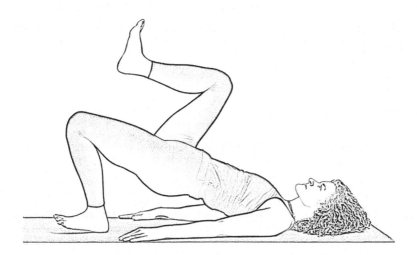

6.  Push the heel into the ground and engage the left buttock. Lift your pelvis 1 to 3 inches. Hold 10–30 seconds, remembering to breathe. You can also coordinate movement and breath (exhale up, inhale down).

7.  Press the fingertips into the left glute and note the firmness. You will compare this feeling when doing the other side.

8.  Come back down to the floor. Repeat on the other side.

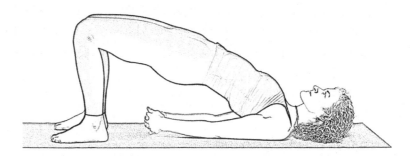

*Note:* When practicing the full Bridge Pose, push the heel of the weaker glute into the floor more firmly. In other words, press the heels asymmetrically to enable symmetrical firing of the glutes.

### Lunge *(Anjaneyasana)*

Preview: This pose was mentioned in the Neutral Pelvis, Neutral Spine section but placed here to focus on whether your glutes are engaged in the back leg. Many students do not engage the back leg buttock and end up putting a lot of pressure on the front of their hip joint.

**Props**

•  Two blocks

•  Optional: blanket to pad the back knee

**How to Practice**

1.  Start in mountain pose with a block close to the outer edge of each foot.

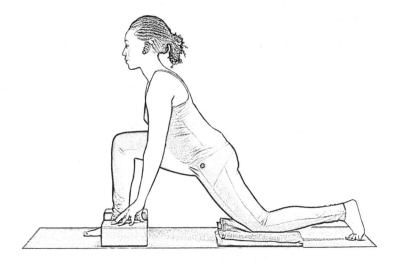

2. Bend forward and place your hands on the blocks (height of the block is determined by you). Keep the hands on the blocks as you step the left foot back into a lunge position. The right knee aligns over the right heel, and the left foot is as far back as it will go. *Note:* This should provide a stretch in the front of the groin or quadriceps of the back (left) leg.

3. Reach through the back heel continuously as you slowly lower the left knee to the floor. Ensure that you maintain the stretch in the front of the back leg. If you lose the stretch, you've stopped reaching through the heel.

4. As you stay in the pose, push through the left heel, while keeping the left knee on the floor. *Note:* Touch the left fingertips to the left buttock and note whether it is engaged. If not, contract your left gluteus maximus. This contraction keeps the left femur aligned and stretches the left groin more. Without this engagement, the femur can push forward into the groin area and, over time, may cause injury.

5. Stay in low lunge for 1–2 minutes.

6. To come out, step the left leg forward next to the right.

7. Repeat on the other side.

## *Clam Shell*

Preview: This pose strengthens the hip abductors, particularly the gluteus medius and minimus. If done correctly, you should feel the muscles around the back of the hip engage when the top leg is lifted. It is crucial that the pelvis be in neutral while in this position. If your lower back rounds, the quadriceps will take over.

### Props

- Optional: blanket for your head
- Optional: elastic exercise band to place around lower thighs

### How to Practice

1. Lie down on your right side so that the hips are stacked with the head supported on your arm or a blanket.

2. Bend the knees 45° so that the heels are in line with the pelvis. *Note:* It is very important that the pelvis be anteriorly tilted in this position. In other words, stick your butt out.

3. Keep the inner edges of the heels touching. Using real or imagined resistance, slowly lift the right knee away from the left as much as you can without rounding the lower

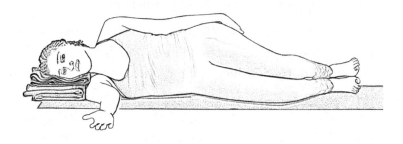

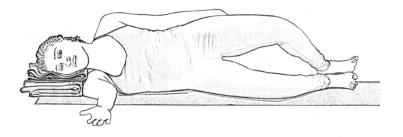

back. *Note:* If you are doing it correctly, you should feel the gluteus minimus and outer thigh activating.

4.  Lower the leg slowly. Do three sets of 10–15 repetitions.

5.  Turn onto the left side and repeat.

**Modification**

*   If there is pain or weakness in the upper leg when lifting, place a pillow or folded blankets between the knees to make the pose more accessible. The most challenging part of this pose is the initial lift, so this helps give you a head start.

*   To make this more challenging, you can place an elastic band around the lower thighs to increase resistance.

A common challenge in lateral standing poses (triangle, warrior 2, extended side angle) is having too much weight in the front foot and not enough in the back foot. When there is too much weight in the front leg, the front hip and back groin can be strained.

One of the reasons this happens is insufficient engagement of the back leg's gluteus. Ideally, all three gluteus muscles of the back leg are engaged: the maximus aids in hip extension; the medius and minimus aid in external rotation of the femur. Without enough muscular engagement in the back glutes, the back foot often collapses onto its inside edge. Or students sickle the ankle bone to avoid collapsing the back arch. The back foot should press evenly into the floor, with the inner and outer heel grounded and the ball of the foot pressing into the floor so that the inner arch lifts.

To activate the gluteus muscles in these poses, bend the back leg knee and externally rotate the thighbone and knee by engaging the gluteus, particularly the gluteus medius and minimus. External rotation of the thighs helps to bring the pelvis into more of a posterior tilt. **This is what you want for these poses!** Keep the buttocks engaged and firm, slowly straightening the back leg. You might feel that your buttocks work more than you are used to. In triangle pose, you can do this with both legs at the same time.

These "Hey, I finally get to tuck" poses activate buttocks, pelvic floor, and legs more than you might be used to. Working this way in standing poses helps your stability. When you feel more stable, the body works more efficiently and your breath should be deeper.

### *Warrior 2 (*Virabhadrasana 2*)*

Preview: The renderings show the pose and the action of bending the back leg to get more rotation on the back leg and firmer in the buttock. This pose will work the feet and engage the inner thighs right up to the perineum. In this version, we'll focus more on the work of the back leg buttock.

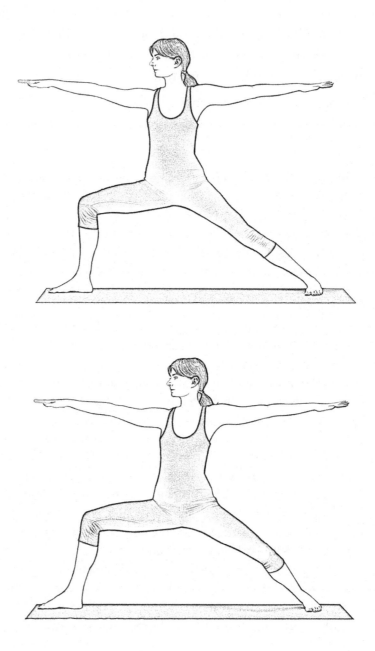

**How to Practice**

1. Begin in mountain pose.

2. Step the feet wide apart, 4–5 feet. Align the heels.

3. Turn the right thigh and foot out 90°.

4. Pivot the left foot slightly inward but turn the left thighbone outward. As the thigh turns out, the left buttock should become firm.

5. Lift through the arches of the feet. Root down through the heels.

6. Keep the external rotation of both thighbones and bend both knees to help externally rotate the thighs more. The buttocks will engage more in response.

7. Keep the extra external rotation and engagement of the buttocks that you gained from bending the knees as you slowly straighten both legs for a moment.

8. Raise the arms to shoulder height out to the sides so they are parallel to the floor and aligned directly over the legs. With the palms facing down, reach actively from fingertip to fingertip.

9. Press down through the inner and outer edges of the back foot and keep the back leg straight with quadriceps and kneecap lifted.

10. On an exhalation, bend the front knee. Align it directly over the ankle of the front heel. The front shin should be perpendicular to the floor. Bring the front thigh as parallel to the floor as you are able.

11. Keep the torso perpendicular to the floor, with the crown of the head directly over the perineum.

12. Turn the head to gaze out across the tip of the right middle finger. Broaden the collarbones. Drop the shoulders. Lift the chest.

13. Draw the sides of the navel in toward the spine and lift the front hip points toward the ribcage.

14. Hold for up to 1 minute.

15. To release, inhale as you press down through the back foot and straighten the front leg. Lower the arms.

16. Turn to the left, reversing the position of the feet, and repeat for the same length of time on the opposite side.

### Modifications

• If balance is a challenge, do the pose in front of a wall with your back to the wall. Alternatively, you can have a chair in front of you and hold the chair while doing the leg actions.

### Focused Actions

• You will feel the pelvic floor muscles activate more when you strongly push down through the inner and outer heels and externally rotate the legs more. Remember, external rotation of the thighbones contracts the pelvic floor muscles.

### *Extended Side Angle (*Uttitha Parsvakonasana*)*

Preview: This pose is essentially deepening the actions of warrior 2. This pose demands even more from the back leg and buttock and adds a side extension. The instructions are the same as for warrior 2 pose up to instruction 10 and they build from there. This pose will work the feet and engage the inner thighs right up to the perineum. In this version, we'll focus more on the work of the back leg buttock.

### Prop

• Block

### How to Practice

1. Begin in mountain pose.

2. Step the feet wide apart, 4–5 feet. Align the heels.

3. Turn the right thigh and foot out 90°.

4. Pivot the left foot slightly inward but turn the left thighbone outward. As the thigh turns out, the left buttock should become firm.

5. Lift through the arches of the feet. Root down through the heels.

6. Keep the external rotation of both thighbones and bend both knees to help externally rotate the thighs more. The buttocks will engage more in response.

7. Keep the extra external rotation and engagement of the buttocks that you gained from bending the knees as you slowly straighten both legs for a moment.

8. Raise the arms to shoulder height out to the sides so they are parallel to the floor and aligned directly over the legs. With the palms facing down, reach actively from fingertip to fingertip.

9. Press down through the inner and outer edges of the back foot and keep the back leg straight with quadriceps and kneecap lifted.

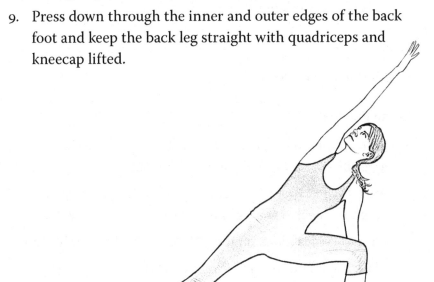

10. On an exhalation, bend the front knee. Align it directly over the ankle of the front heel. The front shin should be perpendicular to the floor. Bring the front thigh as parallel to the floor as you are able.

11. Then, maintaining the stability of your left (back) leg, bring your right forearm to your right thigh or your right hand to a block on the outside of the right foot (more challenging).

12. If you feel that you have lost some of the weight in the back foot, re-bend your back leg and try for more external rotation of the back thigh and engagement of the back leg buttock. Slowly re-straighten the left leg.

13. To come out, push into the left foot on an exhalation and straighten your bent leg.

### Triangle Pose (Trikonasana)

Preview: This pose, when performed properly, encourages active engagement of the pelvic floor muscles, especially through the positioning and work of the legs.

**Props**

• Optional: one block

**How to Practice**

1. Start in mountain pose. On an exhale, separate the feet 3–3.5 feet, a bit more if you have long legs.

2. Turn the left foot in 45°. Turn the right foot and leg out 90°. Align the heel of the right foot with the heel of the left.

3. Place the yoga block on the outside edge of the right shin.

4. Place the hands on the hips and feel the weight in the feet. Keep more weight in the heels and more weight in the back foot.

5. Bend both knees to help externally rotate the thighs. The buttocks will engage more in response. Keep the extra

external rotation and engagement of the buttocks that you gained from bending the knees as you slowly straighten the legs.

6. Strongly contract the quadriceps muscles to stabilize the knee joints.

7. Raise the arms to shoulder height out to the sides so they are parallel to the floor and aligned directly over the legs. With the palms facing down, reach actively from fingertip to fingertip.

8. Keeping the back leg anchored by pressing the inner and outer heel of the left foot to the floor, exhale and extend the torso to the right, directly over the plane of the right leg. *Note:* Bend from the hip joint, not the waist.

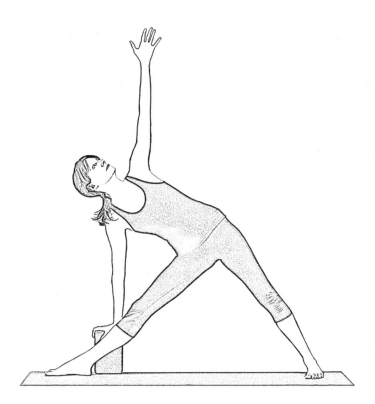

9. Keep the external rotation of the right leg. Ground the right inner heel and ball of the foot into the floor. Bring the front leg sitting bone toward the perineum.

10. Place the right hand on the block. Stretch the left arm toward the ceiling.

11. Keep the head in a neutral position so that the neck is in line with the spine.

12. Remain in this pose for 1 minute.

13. To come out of the pose, strongly press the back heel into the floor and raise the torso.

### Modifications

• Reverse the feet and repeat the pose for the same length of time to the left.

• If you have long legs or tight hamstrings (or both) use a chair for your front hand. It is more important to stay grounded in the legs than to get lower to the ground.

### *Dynamic Chair Pose Using a Chair (*Utkatasana*)*[4]

Preview: This pose helps strengthen the legs, bring awareness to imbalances in your legs, and find assistance from your pelvic floor when sitting down and standing up in yoga practice and real life.

### Props

• Folding chair, or dining chair with a firm, level seat

• Block for between the calves

• Optional: second block to be used between the thighs right above the knees. This prevents the knees and inner arches of the feet from collapsing inward.

**How to Practice**

1. Sit on the chair with the sitting bones in the middle of the seat. *Note:* Do not sit all the way toward the back of the chair.

2. Place the feet flat on the floor so that the shins are perpendicular to the floor. *Note:* You may need to start with the feet closer to the chair so that standing up from sitting will be more accessible, but keep in mind you want to work toward shins starting perpendicular to the floor.

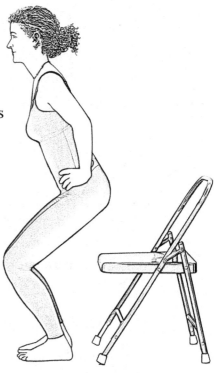

3. Place a block between the lower legs. The face of the block is held by the inner calves.

4. Place the hands on the hips.

5. Push into the heels and keep the torso as upright as possible as you come to standing.

6. Reverse the process and sit down. *Note:* As you go to sit back into the chair, make sure you're sticking the tailbone out. This engages the glutes.

**Modifications**

- To make this more challenging, slow down the process of sitting down and standing up.

### *Dynamic Mountain Pose (*Tadasana*) and Chair Pose (*Utkatasana*) Not Using a Chair*

Preview: The difference between this and the previous pose is that you use this exercise to shift between having weight in the heels and having weight in the balls of the feet. Notice the hamstrings and glutes work when the weight is in the heels. Conversely, the quadriceps work when the weight is in the balls of the feet.

**How to Practice**

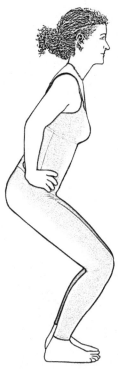

1. Start in mountain pose, hands on hips.

2. Keep more weight in the heels than in the balls of the feet.

3. On an exhale, bend the knees and move the buttocks back as if you were going to sit in a chair. *Note:* It is important to stick your tail out! This makes the buttocks and hamstrings work as opposed to the quads. If you let the tail tuck, it transfers the work into the front of the leg.

4. Maintaining the natural curves of the spine, keep the torso perpendicular to the floor (minimize tipping the upper body forward).

5. Remain in this pose for 30 seconds trying to work up to 1 minute.

6. To come out, on an exhalation, push into the heels, lift the inseam of the thighs toward the perineum, then lift the perineum to engage the pelvic floor. Straighten the legs to return to mountain pose.

**Modification**

• The hamstrings and buttocks will work more the closer you get to a 90° angle between thighs and calves. But when doing this pose in the middle of the room, you are limited in how close you can bring the legs to 90°. Holding onto a kitchen sink, yoga ropes, or a secured banister, bend the knees so that the shins are perpendicular to the floor and the thighbones are parallel to the floor. Make sure that you're not tucking your tail. Pressing weight into the heels, alternate bending and straightening the legs. Repeat 5–10 times.

### *Downward Facing Dog (***Adho Mukha Svanasana***)*

Preview: In the hypertonic section, we bent the legs so that we could stretch the pelvic floor muscles without tight hamstrings getting in the way. This version with straight legs targets a stretch to the buttocks and hamstrings.

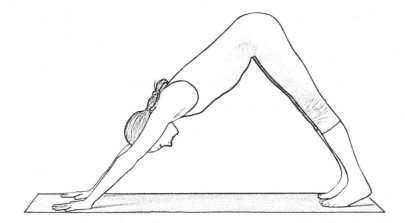

**How to Practice**

1.  Come onto the hands and knees with the hands a whole hand length (about 6 inches) forward of the shoulder joints. The hips should be directly over the knees with the pelvis in an untucked position as in cow.

2.  Spread the fingers and ground down into the hands, especially into the thumb mound and root of the index finger.

3.  Tuck the toes and lift the knees off the floor. Strongly pull the hips away from the hands. Extend through the tail and sitting bones, lifting them toward the ceiling. Pushing into the balls of the feet, stretch the heels away from the toes (think heels back, not down). Focusing on heels down rounds the back.

4.  Push the thighbones back by engaging the quadriceps and draw the pelvis away from the torso, straightening the legs to start.

5.  Keep the ribcage stable—don't be a rib-poker-outer!

6.  Keep the ears in line with the inner arms.

7.  Rotate the thighs inward and keep pushing the hips up toward the ceiling and away from the arms.

8.  Stay in the pose for 20 seconds to 2 minutes.

9.  To come out, bend the knees and rest in child's pose.

### Modifications

- If this pose is challenging to hold, you can elevate your hands on yoga blocks (or on a chair placed against a wall or on the wall itself). This will help take some weight out of the shoulders.

### *Figure Four Pose*

Preview: If the previous pose is too intense, this pose offers a gentler stretch of the same muscle group.

### Props

- Optional: strap or block

### How to Practice

1.  Lie on the back, knees bent, feet on the floor.

2.  Draw the right thigh into the chest.

3.  Turn the right thighbone out.

4.  Place the right ankle above the left knee.

5.  Flex the right ankle.

6.  For a deeper stretch, bring the left foot off the floor and draw the left thigh toward the chest. Bring the right arm through the legs and interlace the hands either behind the left thigh or around the front of the left shin.

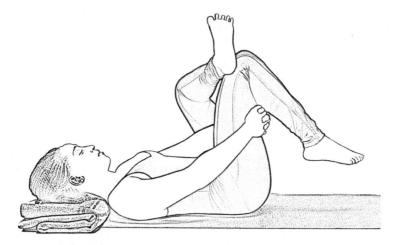

7. Your weight may shift toward one side as you perform this pose. Keep the weight evenly distributed on the back of the pelvis and more toward the top of the sacrum than the bottom. Hold for 1–2 minutes.

8. Change sides.

### Modifications

- If you cannot reach your thigh to draw the legs toward the chest, place a strap around the back of the bottom thigh and pull on the strap to bring your legs up. Or, instead of the strap, place a block under the bottom foot at any height.

# v | Changing the World: One Pelvis at a Time

Big shifts or events often happen instantaneously, but it may also take a long time to get things to that point. Often, the pressure builds slowly. Subterranean rumblings vibrate for a long time, then something happens: a slight movement in the tectonic plates and, all of a sudden an unexpected energy bursts forth, ushering in something new and unforeseen. Such a process describes how I came to teach about the magical female pelvis and finally to write this book. I hope such welcome and transformative shifts will happen for you.

My students had been asking me to put this book together for years, but each time I got started, something always happened to push it into the background. Besides, I couldn't quite believe that it was possible for me to write a book like this, even with its imperfections. One night, I had a wondrous dream, a sign that things were about to change.

In this dream, I was inside a familiar place. The place felt like a compilation of the many homes I had grown up in. Night was about to fall and I heard rustling outside my bedroom. Warily walking toward the window, I almost tripped over my old, tattered suitcase. As I bent down to move it, a tarantula with bright orange and black stripes on its furry legs crawled out. My first impulse was to kill her. But I was struck by her beauty, so I decided that catch and release was a better option. I searched for something to contain her with, but when I came back, she was gone.

The restless, rustling sound continued outside. This time, I walked up to the window and looked through it, and there I saw a great windstorm in the yard. A mass of brown twigs was being whirled about. As I watched the twigs dance, to my amazement, they started taking form. I watched as the twigs took the form of a gorilla. The gorilla approached the window, but somehow I knew that this was not some wild and dangerous beast. On the contrary, I was mesmerized by the love I felt emanating from him. He had beautiful blue eyes and we just stared at one another through the window. This was when the gorilla telepathically explained to me how much love there was in the world. He gestured for me to go across the bedroom and look out the other window. In my dream, I knew that on the other side of the house was a small fountain. But when I looked out the opposite window, it was no longer an ordinary fountain—atop the fountain was a statue of Lakshmi, the Hindu goddess of abundance and prosperity. No longer filled with just water, the entire fountain basin overflowed with blooming flowers. The colors were vibrant, varied, and bursting with beauty.

I immediately left the house to be closer to the flowers. The night sky was bright. I looked up expecting to see a full moon. My eyes fixed on a large glowing object, but as I stared, I realized the orb of a streetlight had tricked me. As much as I searched, I couldn't find the moon. As I lowered my gaze, my partner suddenly appeared beside me. He took my hand and pointed to the sky: "There she is," he whispered, "waxing . . . it won't be long till she's full." And there, in the dark velvet of the night, I saw it: a perfect half moon.

I awoke from this dream intensely happy. I wasn't sure what it all meant, but I knew it was good. I began to research dream symbols, talk to friends, and search within myself for what the deeper meaning might be. Since I've always loved tarantulas, and I believe this one was a "she," I interpreted the tarantula as a symbol of my feminine creative force. It crawled out of my old suitcase and wandered off in a new direction. The gorilla gazing at me with complete acceptance and love bid me to look at my wild, sexual nature without fear and judgment. And the basin of the pool overflowing with bright flowers was a vivid image of abundance (remember, *pelvis* means "basin" in Latin). My search for the full moon (a classic symbol of feminine energy) and my discovery of the waxing half moon stood for my growth, manifestation, and attainment.

Within days of having the dream, I talked to my partner about my neglected book idea. As he did in my dream, he took my hand and said, "Look, the book is already half done, you can finish it." And with that, I began to work on it.

My deepest hope, dear reader, is that this book will point you toward something that inspires you, lights you up, and sparks hope and curiosity in you. My wish is that this book be something that you draw strength and confidence from—just as I did from my dream. And just as my dream showed me love and acceptance, I want you to discover and cultivate a positive and loving relationship with your body. With all the evidence out there, how can we not question "the norm" and push back on popular culture? If nothing else, I hope this book makes you knowledgeable—and proud—of this fascinating part of the female body. Let's bring this topic into mainstream conversation without guilt, shame, or fear. Let's recalibrate our inner dialogue to have compassion for ourselves. Our bodies are truly magical works of art that we should talk to and understand, nourish and celebrate.

By the time you read these words, I hope you have written down the story of your pelvis, and that you have begun to see more clearly the factors impacting your pelvic health. You may have performed internal massages and gained a deeper understanding of the path you need to take for your own healing. You may have begun to walk that path toward new health and self-empowerment. If you are doing these things, I believe that you will come to a very important realization—that you are not alone.

What you will experience has been experienced by millions of women throughout history. To one degree or another, we all face the same conditions and societal factors that contribute to our health challenges. The seeds we are planting for our own awakening are the very same seeds that women have planted for millennia. When we begin to take responsibility and tune into our bodies' innate wisdom, we are tuning into the same power women have experienced since the beginning of time. Lakshmi is the Hindu goddess of prosperity and abundance for all of us. When we begin to awaken to our own potential, it's like entering a flowing river.

It is important to open ourselves and listen to that stream because its currents support us and carry us onward. It may be tempting to complain and feel sorry for all that's happened to us—or worse, to ask ourselves what we did to deserve our misfortunes—but that won't help. It decreases our potential for healing and increases our sense of isolation. Rather, we can cultivate compassion and wisdom, knowing that these elements are older and bigger than we are.

Every pose or posture we take carries energy we can tap into. Every breath brings a sense of aliveness we can feel if we tune in. Sometimes, we can stop negative self-talk by simply changing our posture. We need to stop treating our bodies like the enemy, stop believing the all-pervasive message that we are not good enough. We simply need to listen. When we feel our feet on the ground, our hands on our belly, and our breath flowing through us, we are in sync with a force that's more powerful than even the most sophisticated marketing machine.

Let's make our pelvis, and the miraculous body that houses it, a topic of conversation among our friends and in our community. Sharing is a gift of friendship, and being vulnerable to a friend or family member about what you are going through is an act of strength. Conversely, listening to a friend or a family member not only gives relief to that person, it also builds deeper intimacy in our relationships. Listening is an act of love, and love creates community.

Every now and then, we all need a big gorilla to encourage us with love and compassion through our struggles, to show us the way to the overflowing garden of abundance. And we need somebody to hold our hand and point us in the right direction, so we can trust ourselves to wax into full brightness.

I know how yoga and breathing practices have supported and empowered me in this process. They have helped me to not only overcome pelvic pain, but to better understand my body and to create a healthier relationship with it. The healthier our relationship to our bodies, the happier we are. This, in turn, affects the people in our lives and the community at large. So am I really saying that by liberating our pelvis from pain and suffering, we can make the world a better place? Yes, I am. Together we can change the world, one pelvis at a time.

# APPENDIX
## Where to Go from Here:
## How You Can Use This Book with a Group

If this book has touched you, if it has annoyed you, inspired you, taught you, or if it has raised questions or at least made you curious, my hope is that you will take those sentiments out into the world and share them. The subject of female pelvic health has been shrouded in clouds of secrecy and spoken of in hushed voices for too long. Imagine a world where we can talk about pelvic challenges openly and freely, without fear or embarrassment, maybe even with laughter and fun. One of my goals in writing this book was to help start the conversation, and I cannot think of a better way for any of us to do that than by talking to our friends and other women interested in the subject. Let's get into the driver's seat and start forming our own personal groups. Let's share, inspire each other, explore together, and support one another.

When you consider forming or joining a group, follow Kant's wise counsel to make it no smaller than the number of Graces (three), and no larger than the number of Muses (nine). You can start by simply asking yourself: Are there women in my life who I think would appreciate reading this book? Are there women in my life who I would like to talk with? Is there a pelvic floor yoga teacher in my community I could tap? Are there people in my yoga studio who might be interested?

Getting together with a group is a sure way to up your game. Here are three tacks a group might take:

1.  Discuss the book or individual topics in the book.

2. Explore, share, and discuss personal pelvic history, challenges, and rewards.

3. Discuss and practice pelvic health yoga together.

Let's take a look at each of these options.

**Option 1:** Start your group conversation by asking what ideas in the book people found surprising, interesting, inspiring, or controversial. I venture to guess that before long, you will have a good discussion going. Or you can choose a chapter or topic you are particularly interested in and have everybody read the corresponding sections of the book before diving in.

Whichever way you proceed, here are a few possible discussion points you might consider:

- The book is written by a woman from a white, middle class, East Coast American background who has also lived in the San Francisco Bay Area for over 20 years. Obviously, this background informs her views. Do you relate culturally, or has your experience been shaped by different influences? What discrepancies and similarities in backgrounds do you perceive? How have the differing cultural, social, and emotional experiences of the individuals in your group affected your differing relationships to your bodies?

- Do you share the author's cultural critiques? Do you agree with her views of the challenges women need to overcome? If so, what do you think are the best ways to go about solving these challenges?

- Have you learned from the book or have you been inspired in ways that have led you personally to change? How?

**Option 2:** Our pelvises and our pelvic histories are storehouses of emotion. Let's explore together and share: there is a lot we can learn from each other.

Most sections in the first two chapters of the book have pelvic inquiry sections. Reflect on these questions in private, write down your findings, and then share with a group what you feel comfortable sharing.

Sharing our own story in a group can be very powerful. It can also make us feel vulnerable. As a group, agree in advance on guidelines that will facilitate supportive listening and discussion. For example, you may want to set a time limit for the sharing, and you may want to clarify upfront what responses, if any, are considered helpful. We have to ensure that we support each other and not do more harm.

- What situations trigger awareness of your relationship to your pelvis (and your body)? How does that relationship affect you in general and on a day-to-day basis?

- How have you been trying to change that relationship? What successes have you had? Why do you think what you've tried has worked or not worked?

- How can we support each other in gaining a healthy and joyful relationship to our pelvises and to our bodies?

**Option 3:** I encourage everybody to have a private yoga practice (if possible, daily). Practicing with a friend or in a group can be tremendously helpful. Yoga classes are great, but when we practice with friends we can correct each other's poses, chat and laugh in between poses, and tailor our practice exactly to fit our needs.

Particularly when we practice with other women who are also interested in exploring pelvic health issues, we can discuss the specific pelvic health issues we are working on and then practice together, alternating talk and practice exploration. This allows us not only to learn from each other, but also to have a lot of fun along the way.

∼

There is no limit to our imaginations, individually and collectively. Maybe you want to mix up your book group with a party? How about a vulva- or uterus-themed art party? Think maps, photographs, paintings, food, apparel, music, films . . . I invite you to be daring and creative. Expand your thinking. Grow your limits. In the (slightly altered) words of Margaret Mead: "Never doubt that a small group of daring, powerful women can change the world; indeed, it's the only thing that ever has."

# POSE SEQUENCES

The following pages contain some suggested sequences. Go slow and see what works for you, as everyone's pelvis is different. The first group of poses is to help alleviate hypertonic pelvic floor or pelvic pain. Try this sample sequence for a week and then add the second group of poses one at a time. If you notice that any particular pose aggravates you, delete it from the sequence, then look through the hypertonic section, and slowly add new poses.

Eventually as your tightness and pain subside, try adding a few poses from the hypotonic section but always remember to end your session with a pose or two that you know works for you as a release, followed by *shavasana*.

## Hypertonic Pelvic Floor, Sample Sequence

This sample sequence is for those of you who have a hypertonic pelvic floor or pelvic pain. Try the sample sequence for a week, then add more poses depending on how much time and energy you have.

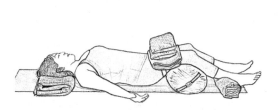

Relaxation Pose with Weight (*Shavasana*)
*page 120*

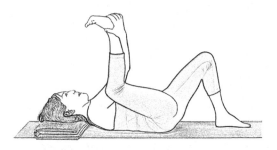

Half Happy Baby Pose (*Ardha Ananda Balasana*) *page 137*

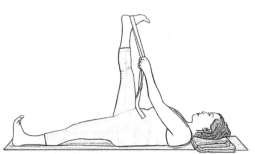

Reclining Big Toe Pose 1
(*Supta Padagushthasana* 1) *page 131*

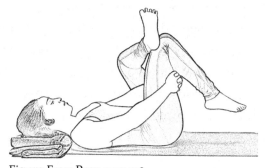

Figure Four Pose *page 218*

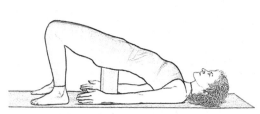

Supported Bridge Pose
(*Setu Bandhasana Sarvanghasana*) *page 158*

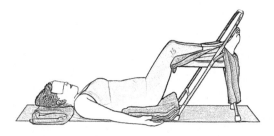

Legs on Chair (*Viparita Karani Mudra*)
*page 163*

## *After a Week, Slowly Add These Poses (in This Order)*

Tail Wag

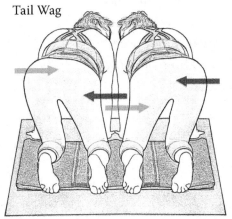

Dynamic Tabletop (Tail Wag) *page 140*

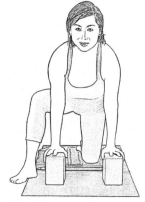

Lunge with Circular Movement 1
(*Anjaneyasana* Variation 1)
*page 145*

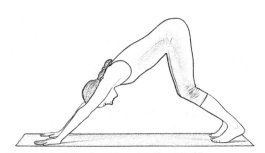

Downward Facing Dog (*Adho Mukha Svanasana*) *page 146*

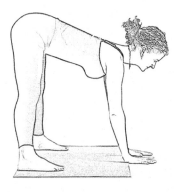

Wide-Legged Standing Forward Bend Pose
(*Prasarita Padottanasana*) *page 152*

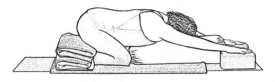

Child's Pose (*Balasana*) *page 143*

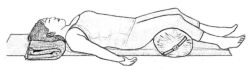

Corpse Pose (*Shavasana*) *page 164*

## Hypotonic Pelvic Floor, Sample Sequence

This sample sequence is for those of you who know you need to strengthen and tone your pelvic floor. Try the sample sequence for a week and then add more poses depending on how much time and energy you have.

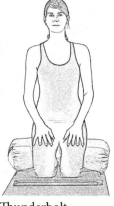

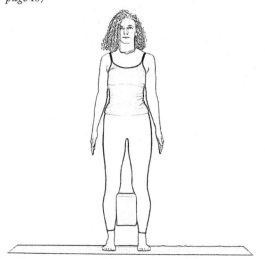

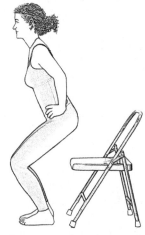

Relaxation Pose with Weight (*Shavasana*)
*page 167*

Thunderbolt
(*Vajrasana*) *page 186*

Mountain Pose (*Tadasana*)
with Block between Inner Legs *page 170*

Dynamic Chair Pose Using a Chair
(*Utkatasana*) *page 214*

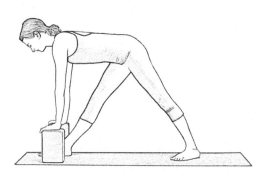

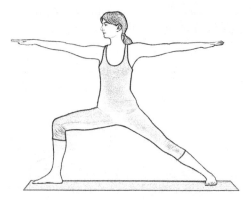

Intense Side Stretch Pose (*Parshvottanasana*)
*page 171*

Warrior 2 (*Virabhadrasana* 2) *page 178*

## *After a Week, Slowly Add These Poses (in This Order)*

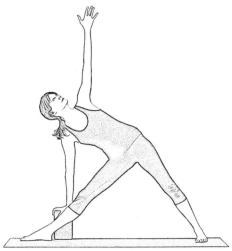

Triangle Pose (*Trikonasana*) *page 212*

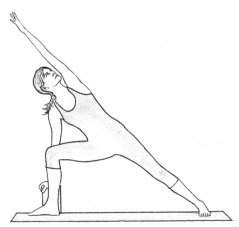

Extended Side Angle
(*Uttitha Parsvakonasana*) *page 210*

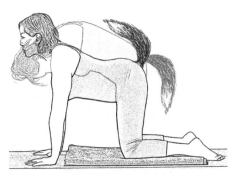

Tabletop, Cat-Cow *page 183*

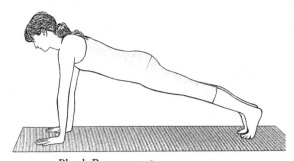

Plank Pose *page 184*

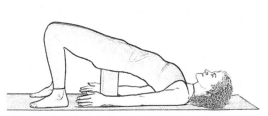

Supported Bridge Pose
(*Setu Bandhasana Sarvanghasana*) *page 193*

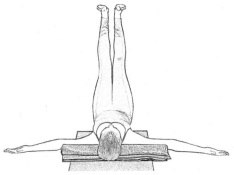

Legs Up the Wall Pose (*Viparita Karani*
Variation) *page 202*

# ACKNOWLEDGMENTS

I feel so much gratitude for the love and support of the many, many dear friends, dedicated professionals, and teachers without whom this book would not have come into being. This book would not have been possible without the proverbial village that it took to birth it.

A big shout out to Dale Casale and Joanna Frueh for starting the whole damn thing. And an even bigger thanks to Jürgen Möller whose brilliant organizing skill and content-development helped shape a very disorganized mess of thoughts into something that looked like a book.

Immense thanks, to my photo editor Sylvia Cruz, WWNYC, without whose help this book would have no asana.

To Avery Kalapa and her incredible talent at understanding what I was trying to convey and somehow making it real through illustrations that make my tail wag.

Thank you for your smart and sassy editing, Shalmali Pal, Lucy Smith, and Bill Anelli. I appreciate how you showed love, precision, and occasional ruthlessness with the red pen.

I feel deep appreciation toward my beautiful and patient yoga models, Margi Young, Kaleen Woo, and Elizabeth Ohito.

Thank you to my early readers, Katherine Lindeburg, Laura Paull, Holly Holt, Shana Chrystie, and Cheryl Ishida for your important feedback.

Thank you, Katarzyna Kopańska for making endlessly beautiful artwork of the female body and making my cover possible.

Profound thanks goes to Susanne Kemmerer for introducing me to my pelvic floor. And to my pelvic floor goddesses and physical therapists Amy Selinger, Isa Herrara, and especially Lizanne Pastore. Lizanne's guidance along the path to healing my own very unhappy pelvis, as well as her input on the anatomical descriptions used in this book, are deeply appreciated.

My gratitude goes to Leslee Subak and Alison Huang at UCSF for inviting me to help design studies demonstrating that yoga can alleviate pelvic floor issues. To Judith Lasater, who I want to be like when I grow up. To Richard Rosen for his endless patience and encouragement on this journey of book writing.

Big *namaste* to my first yoga teacher, Nancy Vinik. Thank you, Nancy, for introducing me to the practice of yoga. And thank you to all of the teachers that have come before you in the lineage of this deep and magical practice.

Immeasurable gratitude to all my teachers and my teachers' teachers, but a special shout out to Swami Ramananda, Rodney Yee, Tony Briggs, Ramanand Patel, Manouso Manos, Patricia Walden, Peter Thompson, Sarah Kotzamani, and (again) Judith Lasater, for your tireless hours of life-changing instruction.

And deeply heartfelt thanks to all of the pelvises that have attended my classes, trainings, and workshops, who have shared their sorrow, pain, joys, and triumphs over the years and have encouraged me to get this book done.

And finally, my profound love and gratitude to Marc Tognotti whose inexhaustible enthusiasm, encouragement, and endless help on this project made something that seemed insurmountable and merely a dream into a reality. You are my full moon.

# NOTES

## Preface

1. Alison J. Huang, Hillary E. Jenny, Margaret A. Chesney, et al. A group-based yoga therapy intervention for urinary incontinence in women: a pilot randomized trial. *Female Pelvic Medicine and Reconstructive Surgery* 2014, 20;3:147–154.

## Chapter I

1. Related reading: Gerda Lerner. 1986. *The Creation of Patriarchy.* Oxford University Press. Barbara Ehrenreich and Deirdre English. 1972. *Witches, Midwives, and Nurses.* The Feminist Press.

2. Laura Stampler. France Just Banned Ultra-Thin Models. Time Newsfeed, Apr 03, 2015. time.com/3770696/france-banned-ultra-thin-models/, accessed July 5, 2017.

3. Doreen Gateless, John Gilroy. Tight-Jeans Meralgia: Hot or Cold? *Journal of the American Medical Association,* 1984;252(1):42-43. jamanetwork .com/journals/jama/article-abstract/393385, accessed July 5, 2017.

4. Press release, American Society of Plastic Surgeons. New Statistics Reflect the Changing Face of Plastic Surgery. Feb. 25, 2016. plasticsurgery .org/news/press-releases/new-statistics-reflect-the-changing-face-of-plastic -surgery, accessed July 5, 2017.

5. Michelle Castillo. Warning: Tight pants, skinny jeans and Spanx may be hazardous to your health. CBS News. cbsnews.com/news/warning-tight -pants-skinny-jeans-and-spanx-may-be-hazardous-to-your-health/, accessed July 5, 2017.

6. Christopher Ingraham. Our infant mortality rate is a national embarrassment. Washington Post Workblog, Sept. 29, 2014. washingtonpost.com/

news/wonk/wp/2014/09/29/our-infant-mortality-rate-is-a-national-embar
rassment/, accessed July 5, 2017.

7. Marian F. MacDorman, T.J. Mathews, Eugene Declercq. Trends in
Out-of-Hospital Births in the United States, 1990–2012. National Center
for Health Statistics, NCHS Data Brief No. 144, March, 2014. cdc.gov/nchs/
products/databriefs/db144.htm, accessed July 5, 2017.

8. Luz Gibbons, José M. Belizán, Jeremy A. Lauer, et al. The Global
Numbers and Costs of Additionally Needed and Unnecessary Caesarean
Sections Performed per Year: Overuse as a Barrier to Universal Coverage.
World Health Report (2010) Background Paper, No 30, who.int/health
systems/topics/financing/healthreport/30C-sectioncosts.pdf, accessed July 5,
2017.

9. National Center for Health Statistics, FastStats. Births—Methods of
Delivery. Births: Final Data for 2015, table 21. cdc.gov/nchs/fastats/delivery
.htm, accessed July 5, 2017.

10. The Hysterectomy Association. Surgical operations and procedures
performed in hospitals—Hysterectomy, by country, 2003–2014. hysterecto
my-association.org.uk/hysterectomy-statistics/, accessed July 5, 2017.

11. National Women's Health Network. Hysterectomy information page,
updated 2015. nwhn.org/hysterectomy/, accessed July 5, 2017.

12. Lauren E. Corona, Carolyn W. Swenson, Kyle H. Sheetz, et al. Use of
Other Treatments before Hysterectomy for Benign Conditions in a Statewide
Hospital Collaborative. *American Journal of Obstetrics & Gynecology*, 2015,
212(3): 304.e1–304.e7. sciencedirect.com/science/article/pii/S0002937814023
552, accessed July 5, 2017.

13. http://www.hersfoundation.com/effects.html.

14. William H. Masters and Virginia E. Johnson. 1966. *Human Sexual
Response*. Boston, MA: Little, Brown.

15. Recommended reading: Jeanne Achterberg. 1990. *Woman as Healer*.
Boston, MA: Shambhala Publications.

16. Barbara Ehrenreich and Deirdre English. 1972. *Witches, Midwives, and
Nurses*. New York, NY: The Feminist Press.

17. ibid.

18. Amy J.C. Cuddy, Caroline A. Wilmuth, and Dana R. Carney. The
Benefit of Power Posing *Before* a High-Stakes Social Evaluation. Harvard
Business School Working Paper, No. 13-027, Sept. 2012. dash.harvard.edu/
bitstream/handle/1/9547823/13-027.pdf?sequence=1, accessed June 11, 2017.

## Chapter II

1. Carl Zimmer. Researchers Find Fish That Walks the Way Land Vertebrates Do. *New York Times,* March 24, 2016. nytimes.com/2016/03/25/science/researchers-find-fish-that-walks-the-way-land-vertebrates-do.html?_r=0, accessed July 6, 2017.

2. http://www.mayoclinic.org/healthy-lifestyle/labor-and-delivery/in-depth/episiotomy/art-20047282, accessed July 14, 2017.

3. Sigrun Hjartardottir, Jan Nilsson, Cecilia Petersen, Goran Lingman. The female pelvic floor: a dome—not a basin. *Acta Obstetricia et Gynecologica Scandinavica,* 1997 Jul;76(6):567–571. ncbi.nlm.nih.gov/pubmed/9246965, accessed June 11, 2017.

4. Sandra Cisneros. 2015. *A House of My Own.* New York, NY: Random House.

5. Brian Palmer. The influence of breastfeeding on the development of the oral cavity: a commentary. *Journal of Human Lactation,* 1998;14(2):93–98. brianpalmerdds.com/bfeed_oralcavity.htm, accessed June 11, 2017.

6. Louisa Williams. From Attention Deficit to Sleep Apnea: The Serious Consequences of Dental Deformities. Oct 30, 2009, westonaprice.org/health-topics/dentistry/from-attention-deficit-to-sleep-apnea/, accessed June 11, 2017. Also, International Association of Facial Growth Guidance (Orthotropics). Evidence Based Therapy. orthotropics.org/science_and_research/index.php, accessed June 11, 2017.

7. Wikipedia. Respiratory Rate. 6/6/17. en.wikipedia.org/wiki/Respiratory_rate, accessed June 11, 2017.

8. http://www.cancernetwork.com/melanoma/melanomas-vulva-and-vagina, accessed July 11, 2017.

9. A vaginal dilator is a cylindrical shaped wand usually made out of silicone that can be used to get to places in the pelvic floor that are harder to get at with your fingers. Also, it can help if your fingers get tired.

10. Dov Sikirov. Comparison of straining during defecation in three positions: results and implications for human health. Dig Dis Sci. 2003 Jul;48(7):1201–1205. ncbi.nlm.nih.gov/pubmed/12870773, accessed June 11, 2017.

11. Ryugi Sakakibara, Kuniko Tsunoyama, Hiroyasu Hosoi, et al. Influence of body position on defecation in humans. Wiley Online Library. Jan 11, 2010. onlinelibrary.wiley.com/doi/10.1111/j.1757-5672.2009.00057.x/abstract, accessed June 11, 2017.

12. Note that if you have active skin irritations, a yeast infection, vulvodynia, or vaginismus, you may not want to put anything up against the perineum as this could aggravate the condition. If you have pelvic pain, you

may want to practice deep breathing and self-massage for a few weeks until you can put something against the perineum without pain.

13. Check Chapter IV for step by step instructions of mountain pose (*tadasana*).

14. Note that the position of your pelvis matters here. Elevating your heels (place them on the edge of a folded blanket) and squatting over the mirror will align your pelvis in a more neutral position.

15. Gail did the complete protocol as taught by Dr. Carol Phillips, D.C. in her Dynamic Body Balancing workshops. The mother's sacrum was pulled into the path of the baby by shortened sacrotuberous ligaments. Gail did myofascial releases and cranial sacral therapy on the woman's cranium.

16. Norman Doidge. 2016. *The Brain's Way of Healing*, New York, NY: Penguin Books.

17. orthotropics.com.

18. Spinal shear is defined as "Forces acting perpendicular to the axis of the spine apply a shearing force that tries to slide the components away from their normal axis. Stresses develop in the interior of the structure. If the shear forces are great enough, ligament and disk tears may result as well as shear fractures of the vertebrae." http://medical-dictionary.thefreedictionary.com/shear.

## Chapter III

1. Centers for Disease Control and Prevention (CDC). Prevalence of incontinence among older Americans. Vital and Health Statistics, series 3, number 36, June 2014. cdc.gov/nchs/data/series/sr_03/sr03_036.pdf, accessed June 11, 2017.

2. Mary K. Townsend, Kim N. Danforth, Karen L. Lifford, et al. Incidence and remission of urinary incontinence in middle-aged women. *Am J Obstet Gynecol.* 2007;197(2):167.e1–5. ncbi.nlm.nih.gov/pubmed/17689637, accessed June 11, 2017.

3. Linda Bren. Controlling Urinary Incontinence. FDA Consumer magazine. September–October 2005. in.gov/isdh/files/FDA.pdf, accessed June 11, 2017.

4. The Association for Pelvic Organ Prolapse Support estimates 34 million women globally suffer with POP. http://www.pelvicorganprolapsesupport.org/pelvic-organ-prolapse-help-and-hope/, accessed July 18, 2017. The American Society of Colon and Rectal Surgeons estimates about 25 people per 1 million have rectal prolapse. ASCRS. Rectal prolapse expanded version. fascrs.org/patients/disease-condition/rectal-prolapse-expanded-version, accessed June 13, 2017.

5. Donald G. McNeil. Ask Well: Catching Disease from a Toilet Seat. NY Times Well Blog. June 8, 2015. well.blogs.nytimes.com/2015/06/08/ask-well -what-diseases-can-i-get-from-a-toilet-seat/?_r=0, accessed June 13, 2017.

6. Docs rarely name stuff after themselves; it's usually some society or institution that bestows the name. Also, there are a lot of female-related medical procedures (C-section, Pap smear) that are named after men because, well, only men were allowed to practice medicine for a long time.

## Chapter IV

1. This scenario is based on stories from women who have attended my workshops.

2. Alison J. Huang, Hillary E. Jenny, Margaret A. Chesney, et al. A group-based yoga therapy intervention for urinary incontinence in women: a pilot randomized trial. *Female Pelvic Medicine and Reconstructive Surgery* 2014, 20;3:147–154.

3. According to yoga teacher Richard Rosen, a *vajra* is a thunderbolt. But the instructions for this pose in the *Ghrenda Samhita* say to make the thighs as hard as a diamond, which is an alternative meaning for *vajra*. So it would seem to make sense to call this diamond pose, as the diamond cuts through all other substances, just as *jnana*/knowledge cuts through *avidya*/ignorance.

4. This pose is commonly referred to as chair pose but the literal translation from the Sanskrit is "fierce."

# ABOUT THE AUTHOR

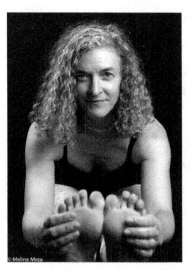

**Leslie Howard** is an Oakland-based yoga teacher, specializing in all things pelvic. Leslie leads Pelvic Floor Yoga certification trainings and other workshops across the United States and internationally. Her teaching is informed by over 3,500 hours of study with senior Iyengar yoga teachers including Manouso Manos, Patricia Walden, and Ramanand Patel. In 2013, Leslie, with contributions from Judith Lasater, co-designed two successful studies at UCSF medical center that demonstrated the effectiveness of her yoga techniques for incontinence and pelvic pain. Leslie's own struggles to heal her hips and pelvis led her to intense study of the anatomy, physiology, cultural messaging, history, and energetics of this complex area of the body. To find out more about Leslie, go to www.pelvicliberation.com.

CPSIA information can be obtained
at www.ICGtesting.com
Printed in the USA
LVOW04s2022241117
557349LV00002B/24/P